Non-Invasive Monitoring of Transdermal Drug Delivery

Non-Invasive Monitoring of Transdermal Drug Delivery

P. Arpaia
U. Cesaro
N. Moccaldi
I. Sannino

CRC Press
Taylor & Francis Group
Boca Raton London New York

CRC Press is an imprint of the
Taylor & Francis Group, an **informa** business

First edition published 2022
by CRC Press
6000 Broken Sound Parkway NW, Suite 300, Boca Raton, FL 33487-2742

and by CRC Press
2 Park Square, Milton Park, Abingdon, Oxon, OX14 4RN

CRC Press is an imprint of Taylor & Francis Group, LLC

Library of Congress Cataloging-in-Publication Data

Names: Arpaia, P. (Pasquale), author. | Cesaro, U. (Umberto), author. | Moccaldi, N. (Nicola), author. | Sannino, I. (Isabella), author.
Title: Noninvasive monitoring of drug bioavailability by tissue impedance measurement / P. Arpaia, U. Cesaro, N. Moccaldi, I. Sannino.
Description: First edition. | Boca Raton : CRC Press, 2022. | Includes bibliographical references and index. | Summary: "The book presents an innovative technology based on injection of a very weak current to trace the quantity of a drug carried immediately after the administration. The book makes the reader familiar with the technology, from the conception through the design of the instrument, up to the preliminary clinical applications"-- Provided by publisher.
Identifiers: LCCN 2021045815 (print) | LCCN 2021045816 (ebook) | ISBN 9780367765989 (hbk) | ISBN 9780367771898 (pbk) | ISBN 9781003170143 (ebk)
Subjects: LCSH: Drugs--Bioavailability. | Nerve tissue.
Classification: LCC RM301.6 .A77 2022 (print) | LCC RM301.6 (ebook) | DDC 615.1/9--dc23/eng/20211105
LC record available at https://lccn.loc.gov/2021045815
LC ebook record available at https://lccn.loc.gov/2021045816

ISBN: 978-0-367-76598-9 (hbk)
ISBN: 978-0-367-77189-8 (pbk)
ISBN: 978-1-003-17014-3 (ebk)

DOI: 10.1201/9781003170143

Typeset in font CMR10
by KnowledgeWorks Global Ltd.

To my father,
for teaching me that there are no bad guys,
but people with reasons I don't understand;
and
to my partner,
for teaching me to smile at idiots,
with reasons I don't understand yet
(perhaps).

Contents

Foreword

This book is an important attempt to let readers to understand the drug bioavailability monitoring. Drugs are important for allowing people to survive the big problems in everyday life, but the drug availability in the body is much more important: we think it is enough to take a pill to have the beneficial effects connected to the drug, but this is not true! What if the pill, which contains a specific drug, is not absorbed by the body?

Monitoring the drug bioavailability is really important and doing such a monitoring in a non-invasive way is vital. The tissue impedance monitoring is based on a non-invasive measurement and this is another important point.

I met one of the authors, Pasquale Arpaia, several years ago. He is a clever researcher with an incredibly high citation number and bibliometric indexes. One of the other authors, Isabella Sannino, is a PhD student in Metrology at Politecnico di Torino and this is something which makes me happy of working for this PhD Course. I also know the work of the other two authors, Umberto Cesaro and Nicola Moccaldi are really connected to the innovation in medical field.

The book contains three case studies belonging to quite many different areas, from Aesthetic Medicine through Diabetology, up to Orthopaedics. It includes an interesting a description of theoretical methods, instruments design criteria, and applications for measurements in such different fields. The methods and the instruments are applied to different subfields: from the aesthetic medicine, namely the hyaluronic acid, through the diabetology, namely the insulin measurement, up to the orthopaedics, namely the knee traumatology.

A very good book, in general, and an important book any researcher in the field should have in his/her library.

Marco Parvis

Former chair of the *IEEE Instrumentation and Measurement Society TC25 on Medical Measurement and Application.*

Preface

This book has an originating reason: my (and of the co-authors) definitive and endless passion for books. As a boy, I inexhaustibly devoured books of all kinds: during summer, the problem was to transport a sufficient quantity of books to our holiday home in Cilento. During other seasons, my father recklessly opened an account for me in the bookshop in front of our home, so that I could buy as many books as I needed. He was immediately forced to close it, because the amount spent in the first months exceeded the budget by at least ten times. I devoured all kinds of novels, at such a speed that several times my uncle, doubting that I could have read the text as a whole, tried to catch me out by opening randomly the book in turn. By reading a passage, he was astonished how I was able to continue perfectly. I have never investigated, but I think I have a particular natural gift of reading several paragraphs in a few seconds. My home before, at the paper age, and my electronic reader now, at the e-books age, are completely flooded with books of all kinds, from scientific texts to historical essays. My family knows how I go subject to periodic passions in which I devour hundreds of related books: the passion for Japan remains proverbial, 300–400 books between essays and literature, or for the Second World War and Fascism, when I have overcome the 500–600 tomes.

Writing such a book arises directly from my passion and that of the co-authors for research. As we approach retirement age, my friends long for the time to hang up one's boots and they complain about how hard their work is turning out to be. I am ashamed to express my point of view: doing research does not weigh on me; namely, I'm ashamed because I get paid to have fun. I inherited this passion for research from my father, a very fine mathematician. Before, he was able to burn the times of the very-severe (at that time) Italian classical high school in one year less. Then, in spite of his humanistic background, he won the ultra-selective competition for being admitted to the Scuola Normale di Pisa in pure mathematics. I also inherited my passion for electrical impedance spectroscopy from him: in preparing a recent keynote lecture, I realized that not only I had been working on this topic for over 25 years, but, moreover, that my father also worked on this topic until his early death. For this reason, I dedicate all the effort that I have playfully produced in this book to him and to his rational kindness.

In times when facts harass opinions, bioimpedance spectroscopy remains a fundamental measurement technique. Not just to distinguish really- from falsely-skinny people. We worked hard until we created an academic spin-off company in aesthetic medicine. The company has survived betrayals of all kinds, from funding agencies to the theft of creative finance. Then, reasonableness we overcame the abyss into which passion plunged us and we abandoned the spin off. The captain is the last to abandon the ship, but sometimes he kicks the bucket. We wanted to survive, perhaps also to tell everything we learned, in Chapters 1, 2, 3, and 7 of this book.

Chapter 1 has an underlying instructive story, such as all the beginnings of important things in our life. In the humble opinion of my white hair, it is one of the best in the book. Indeed, I didn't write it, now a tedious dodderer, nor Nicola Moccaldi, a severe creative researcher. At the end, only the few pages about the instrumentation and the underlying measurement principle were written by Umberto Cesaro, as talented teacher. Isabella Sannino has almost the full authorship of the chapter, despite her initial protests of not being capable at all. She learned that nothing is precluded to those who act with love. Nicola, Umberto, and I, we still have to learn that the youngest pupil can always amaze us. In truth, Umberto Cesaro constantly transcends his technician position with his continuous enthusiasm for work and research. One above all: during last August, in Stromboli, at the beginning of a holiday weekend, I was reached by a phone call from him at dinner. He gave me a faithful report of a session of impedance measurements on eggplants for several minutes, while I was trying in vain to bite a shrimp with spaghetti. I didn't have the heart to stop him, because I was fully seduced by his enthusiasm.

To be fair, the book consists of four stories.

One concerns aesthetic medicine, sketched before, which runs through Chapters 1 (1.2), for the background, 2, on the measurement method, 3, on the relative instrumentation, and 7, about all the work we did before being ready to the clinical trials. Aside from the terrifying but instructive history of the spin-off company, it was an experience full of painful satisfaction. But nothing is better than winning at the end when you before thought to have lost. There, Nicola Moccaldi revealed all his talent for research and a prodigious ability to learn from my mistakes. One of the cornerstones was the publication of the research work on Nature Scientific Report, where we humble experimenters and technologists had never arrived before. One of the most exciting points was moving from eggplant to pig's ears and then to in-vivo tests. Pig ears were a new and somewhat macabre involvement for us, instrumental engineers.

The second story concerns diabetology. Diabetes concerns me closely, as I have a mild form, but it has been present in my family since my childhood, and also now strongly, with my partner. My dear friend Maurizio Taglialatela gave me the idea that we could measure the bioavailability of insulin, during a summer dinner on my terrace in Campo di Mare. I nearly burned the meat on the barbecue. I'm still excited, at least for the research and the barbecue. We then began the new adventure, narrated initially in Chapter 1 (1.3), with the introduction to what we mean by the measurement of diabetes, and then with the description of the method and instrumentation, in Chapters 4 and 5, respectively. Needless to say, the great satisfaction of arriving at the first in-vivo measurements on myself, from the eggplants (not grilled this time) was enormous. Too bad that the research always reserves us with closed doors or cold showers. Isabella Sannino discovered in the preliminary clinic trials that the instrument worked perfectly, but only on me! We rediscovered at the expense of our coronaries that biomedical instrumentation suffers from an immense problem: intra- and inter-individual non-reproducibility. Nicola Moccaldi had a stroke of genius: calibrating the instrument during the injection, in order to have a perfectly personalized model, when the insulin disappears from the injection site, and therefore, triggers bioavailability. Joys and pains of the researcher life. In Chapter 8, the thorough reader will find what we did to get ourselves out of trouble.

The third story is about orthopaedics. To be honest, this story which seems to be the most incomplete, is where we started, or maybe where we wanted to do it. Our entire previous adventure with prosthesis diagnostics is not reported in this book. It began (alas, when I still had black hair) with the generosity of my cousin Vincenzo Bruno, a dentist, of funding a research grant. He had the intuition that we could diagnose osseointegration by impedance spectroscopy. Brilliant intuition, perfectly verified by our subsequent experiments. We then moved on to the related adventure narrated in this book, by generalizing the measures to orthopaedics (Chapter 1, Section 1.4). We then continued with the knee model and its validation with an ad-hoc instrument, described in Chapters 6 and 9, respectively.

And the fourth story? The chapters are finished, the attentive reader tells me, provided that he/she has come this far with me. Well, the fourth story is precisely the story of love for experiments. It runs through the book as a whole, in all its sections. I hope that this love will be projected into the reader's heart and inspire at least a little bit of his/her professional and vital path. Because without love there is no passion, which comes from ancient Greek, and means sufferance. But what satisfaction is there in winning easily? I write these words in Pollica, in my beloved Cilento, on a fiery afternoon at the end of July. I turn around and see Capo Palinuro. In the name of that man, who asleep fell from his boat, and died, after being escaped to 10 years of war, to the massacre of his world, a few steps from his safety. It is not important where we arrive, but how we walk. Here it is the end of the fourth story of this book.

Pasquale "Papele" Arpaia
Pollica, on the 29th of July, 2021.

Acknowledgements

The Authors would like to thank all the people who have helped in working out this book.

First of all, our thanks go to the members of the Laboratory of Augmented Reality for Health Monitoring (ARHeMLab), for their continuous support in the experiments and in revising some book material. It is well known that a cooperative and stimulating environment synergistically multiplies creativity and makes the impossible possible.

We also heartily acknowledge the invaluable help of Domenico Acierno, Melania Allocca, Antonio Aronne, Mario Arpaia Sr., Vincenzo Bruno, Carmine Romanucci, Massimo Clemente, Olfa Kanoun, Rosario Schiano Lo Moriello, Carlo "Massimo" Manna, Maurizio Marvaso, Giuseppe "Lionheart" Montenero, Pasquale Pernice, Giuseppe Principe, Diego Rattazzi, Mirna Urquidi, Renato Torre, Francesco Vicidomini, and Antonio Zanesco for their contribution towards this work.

We would also like to extend our sincere thanks to Marc Gutierrez for his valuable suggestions and encouragement throughout the project.

We are grateful to all the reviewers for their timely review and useful suggestions, which improved significantly the quality, the scientific content, and the readability of the book: Giuseppina Affinito, Aurelio Arpaia, Clelia Dalia, Luigi Duraccio, Antonio Esposito, Ludovica Gargiulo, Francesca Mancino, Giovanna Mastrati, and Ersilia Vallefuoco.

We thank Marco Parvis and Sabrina Grassini, for useful suggestions in Bioimpedance Analysis.

For the research in aesthetic medicine, we thank Pasquale Cimmino, Fernando Coda, and Alessandra Smarra for supporting firmware development and reproducibility tests for impedance measurements, respectively, as well as Mario Ippolito for his experimental support in the in-vivo tests. A special thank is given to Giuseppe Campiani for his capability of detecting intellectual honesty.

For the research in diabetology, we thank prof. Giovanni Annuzzi for stimulating discussions, Maurizio Taglialatela for beneficial conversations and feedback, Dr. Ornella Cuomo for scientific support, Federica Crauso, Mirco Frosolone, and Giovanna Mastrati for help in experiments, during the campaigns with the Insulin Meter, and the Company Eli Lilly for supplying insulin.

For the research in orthopaedics, we thank Simone Minucci and D. Cuneo for the support in building the knee FEM model.

Part of the research was supported by (i) the Italian Ministry of University and Instruction (MIUR), through the Project MATSI (*A Measurement and control system of drug Absorption Transdermal transport therapies by means of Spectroscopy of Impedance*), and (ii) the University of Naples Federico II, through the Project TDeUM (*A Trasdermal Delivery Universal Meter*), whose support the Authors gratefully acknowledge.

We give a special thank to all the bodies and people who, by betraying our trust in others and our innate ability to smile at strangers, by stealing the funds that we have laboriously earned meritocratically, and by treacherously hindering our careers, have contributed to make us stronger and reinforce our good will, main ingredients of our successes, small in the eyes of the world, but immense in our hearts.

Last, but not least, we are indebted to our loved cohabiting and our relatives. They have endured with affection the excesses of our passion, that led us too often to write this book outside working hours, by taking away their precious time. Their patience and support, always delivered with great tact and modesty, helped to enrich and inspire our work, so as to ultimately improve the content and writing of this book.

Author Biographies

Pasquale Arpaia took Master Degree and PhD in Electrical Engineering at University of Napoli Federico II (Italy), where he is full professor of Instrumentation and Measurements. He is Team Leader at European Organization for Nuclear Research (CERN). He was also professor at University of Sannio, scientific associate at Institutes of Engines and Biomedical Engineering of CNR, and now of INFN Section of Naples. He is Associate Editor of the Institute of Physics Journal of Instrumentation, Elsevier Journal Computer Standards & Interfaces, MDPI Instruments, and in the past also of IEEE Transactions on Electronics Packaging and Manufacturing. He was Editor at Momentum Press of the Book Collection "Emerging Technologies in Measurements, Instrumentation, and Sensors". In last years, he was scientific responsible of more than 30 awarded research projects in cooperation with industry, with related patents and international licenses, and funded 4 academic spin off companies. His main research interests include digital instrumentation and measurement techniques for magnets, superconductors, power converters and cryogenics of particle accelerators, evolutionary diagnostics, distributed measurement systems, ADC modelling and testing. In these fields, he published several book chapters, and about 235 scientific papers in journals and national and international conference proceedings. His PhD students were awarded in 2006 and 2010 at IEEE I2MTC, as well as in 2012-2018 and 2016 at IMEKO World and TC-10 Conferences, respectively.

Umberto Cesaro received the M.Sc.Eng. degree in electronic engineering from the University of Naples Federico II, Napoli, Italy. He is currently an Adjunct Professor and a Graduate Engineer with the University of Naples Federico II. His current research interests include digital high-precision instrumentation, ADC modeling and testing, and biomedical instrumentation. In these fields, he published several scientific papers in journals and national and international conference proceedings.

Nicola Moccaldi received the M.Sc. degree (cum laude) in communication science with the Faculty of Arts and Philosophy, University of Salerno, Fisciano, Italy, in 1999, and the B.Sc. degree in electronic engineering, in 2015. Since 1999, he has done numerous professional assignments in the social and health sector policies including: planning and implementation of corporate communication, coordination of complex services, design, and the evaluation of services, on behalf of several nonprofit organizations and government agencies. Since 2015, he joined with university startup (Innovum S.R.L.), as a Researcher in electronic engineering applied to biomedical field. He is currently a Research Fellow with CRdC Tecnologie Scarl, Naples, Italy. His current research interests include biomedical instrumentation and measurement. In this field, he published several scientific papers in journals and national and international conference proceedings.

Isabella Sannino received the M.S. Degree in Biomedical Engineering in 2018. During her Master Thesis she has been working at Cranfield University (England) in Mechatronic Laboratory of Advanced Vehicle Engineering Centre focusing on driver's neuromuscular dynamics. She collaborates with ARHeMLab (Augmented Reality for Health Monitoring Laboratory), part of Department of Electrical engineering and Information Technology. She is currently a Ph.D. student in Metrology at Polytechnic of Turin and her research interests include biomedical instrumentation, bioimpedance and biosignals measurements for biomedical applications.

List of Figures

List of Tables

Introduction

Bioimpedance spectroscopy is considered as a powerful, painless, and harmless measurement method in many medical fields. This book focuses on some applications of bioimpedance spectroscopy in medicine, by paying particular attention to drug bioavailability assessment. As an example, bioimpedance spectroscopy can provide a key support to (i) the evaluation of skin health (aesthetics), (ii) the motivation of people with diabetes to monitor their glucose concentration more frequently (diabetology), and (iii) the diagnostics of the tissues surrounding a prosthesis (orthopaedy).

The potential of transdermal drug delivery is widely appreciated in aesthetic medicine. It guarantees less systemic uptake and no skin irritation with respect to oral administration and hypodermic injection, respectively. However, at present, there are no standardized methods for assessing the amount of drug penetrating the skin during aesthetic treatments. Some precise methods are invasive and burdensome. In case of skin biopsies, a local anaesthesia is needed. "Suction blisters" requires a disruptive pressure on the skin in order to create a sort of bubble with interstitial fluid. The drug is sampled in the blister by a needle and then assessed. Tape stripping is less invasive but requires a progressive removal of layers of stratum corneum. Microdialysis demands the inclusion of a catheter. Other current and auspicious techniques are Confocal Raman spectroscopy and the colorimetry. In the first case, a Raman spectrometer and a standard optical microscope allow to display a highly-magnified sample and the subsequent Raman analysis. However, the necessary devices are very costly, by allowing only the direct analysis of the skin surface.

Diabetes is one of the most spread non-communicable diseases worldwide. Globally, the number of people with diabetes is currently around 400 million and this disease is the fifth leading cause of death in most developed countries, according to the international diabetes federation. For type-1 diabetic patients, monitoring blood glucose concentration and its regulation are crucial issues. The artificial Pancreas (the most recent and advanced solution to support the diabetic patient) consists of glucose sensor control algorithms and an insulin infusion device. The loop is closed in the case of basal insulin administration, meanwhile, in the case of bolus administration, the system cannot react instantaneously to the quick blood glucose variation caused by food ingestion. Therefore, proper algorithms support the patient in the calculation of the bolus dosage by receiving control inputs such as insulin sensitivity factor, and insulin duration of action. They are both subject to relevant variations depending on the kinetics of insulin absorption. Skin alterations, such as lipohypertrophic nodules, are the main causes of intra-individual variability in insulin absorption. These problems affect also advanced automated diabetic therapy. An accurate insulin bolus administration is guaranteed by real-time monitoring of the amount of insulin actually absorbed, namely bioavailable. To date, the main methods for assessing insulin bioavailability are invasive or have high latency.

Knee pain is a particularly common condition; about forty millions of people reporting knee pain, and the incidence increases notably with age. Some of the most common causes are joint or bone injuries, sprains, ligaments strain, tendonitis, or degenerative joint diseases, like osteoarthritis, rheumatoid arthritis, and other inflammatory disorders. The therapy recommended for several of these pathologies often includes topical nonsteroidal anti-inflammatory drug, also known as NSAID. They are effective analgesics, commonly administered by transdermal drug delivery for treating of acute pain and local muscle inflammation. A widely-used approach to improve transdermal drug delivery is iontophoresis. However, at present, there are no acceptable standard methods for exactly assessing the amount of delivered drugs in tissues. This is mainly due to variable (i) intra-individual conditions, such as different body areas, skin conditions, psychological conditions; as well as (ii) inter-individual factors, such as sex, age, ethnicity, and so on. Moreover, currently, the duration of transdermal-delivery-based therapies does not take into account actual individual skin permeability.

In this book, the Authors propose bioimpedance spectroscopy as a non-invasive, low-cost, and in-vivo method for assessing experimentally the bioavailability of drugs. In the case of systemic drugs, bioavailability is typically defined as the rate and amount of drug that reaches the general circulation from an administered dosage. Instead, in the case of topical drugs for local action, bioavailability may coincide with the drug crossing the first layers of the skin. In both the cases, currently, there are no acceptable standard methods for the in-vivo, non-invasive bioavailability assessment. In this book, bioimpedance spectroscopy is proposed as an effective method for the bioavailability assessment of different kinds of drugs with specific reference to aesthetic medicine, diabetology, and orthopaedics.

After the first chapter dedicated to a comprehensive introduction to the use of bioimpedance spectroscopy in medicine, the measurement of the amount of hyaluronic acid penetrated after electroporation in aesthetics medicine is discussed in Chapters 2, 3, and 7. These chapters present a method, an instrument, and a use case, respectively. Chapters 4, 5, and 8 refer to the insulin bioavailability assessment. Again a method, an instrument, and a use case are presented. Finally, Chapters 6 and 9 deal with the development of a Finite Element Model of the knee to improve the measurement accuracy of NSAIDs actually penetrated under the skin after an iontophoresis treatment.

Part I

Background

1

Basic Concepts

CONTENTS

Bioimpedance analysis is considered as a powerful, painless, and harmless method representing a winning choice in many medical fields. In general, measuring a biological impedance requires the injection of an electric current passing through the biological tissue under test. In this chapter, the attention is focused on three different medical fields: aesthetics, diabetology, and orthopaedics.

About the aesthetics, bioimpedance analysis can optimize the assessment of tissue health, improve the differentiation of healthy and carcinogenic tissues, and support anti-aging and miniaturization treatments in skin cosmetics. About the diabetology, the peculiar non-invasiveness of bioimpedance analysis would motivate people with diabetes to monitor their glucose concentration more frequently, or even continuously. In orthopaedics, bioimpedance analysis can be used for diagnosing the outcome of a trauma predictively, for evaluating the health status of bones and joints, monitoring the effect of the drug injection, and assessing the growth state of the tissues surrounding a prosthesis. Finally, in this chapter, the spectroscopy is highlighted as a solution to the relevant bioimpedance problem of using very few analysis frequencies.

DOI: 10.1201/9781003170143-1

1.1 Bioimpedance Measurement Fundamentals

Impedance measurements are essentially based on the voltamperometric method. It relies on measuring the voltage drops across the unknown impedance and a reference standard resistor, both interested by the same current (Fig. 1.1).

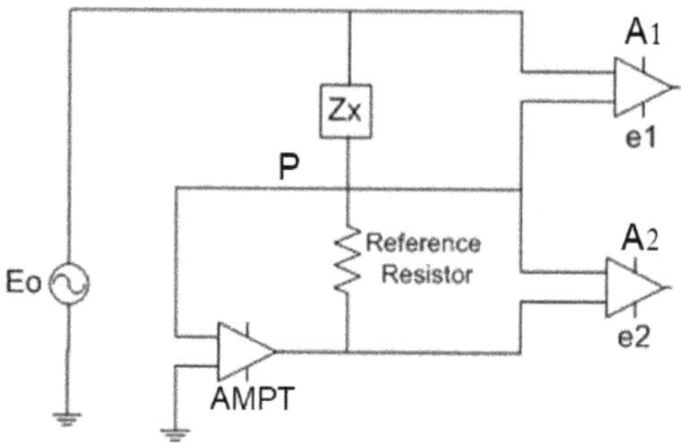

FIGURE 1.1
Elementary voltamperometric circuit for impedance measurement.

The measurement circuit in Fig. 1.1 shows:

- a waveform generator E_o;
- an unknown impedance Z_x;
- a standard reference resistor R_s;
- two differential operation amplifiers A_1 and A_2 used to measure the voltage drop, e_1 and e_2, on the impedance Z_x and on the Reference Resistor, respectively;
- and a transconductance operational amplifier AMPT, to guarantee grounding of the common point P without direct connection (thanks to its virtual mass input).

Different types of impedance meter are available on the market, based on the above voltamperometric method, but differing in the signal processing.

The architecture of a traditional instrument, still useful for educational purpose (GR 1689 RLC Digibridge General Radio®) [1] is shown in Fig. 1.2. In addition to the previously analyzed components, there are:

- a multiplexer (MUX), to connect its single output alternately with the two inputs;

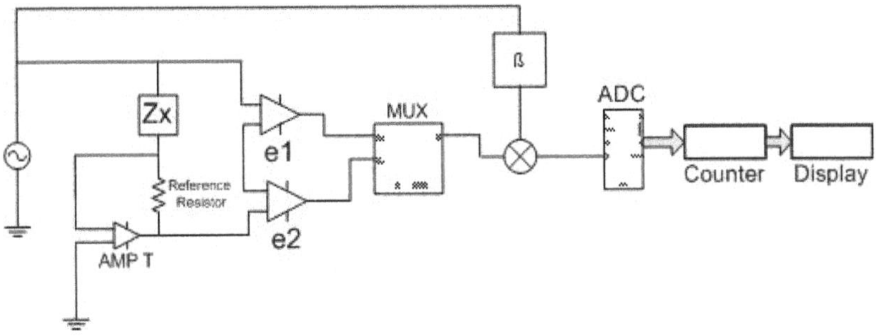

FIGURE 1.2
Block diagram of the impedance meter type General Radio Digibridge® [1].

- an analog multiplier;
- a phase control circuit (named β), which allows to generate signals in or out of phase with the reference by $90°, 180°, 270°$;
- an analog-to-digital converter (typically a double-ramp converter with a voltage-time conversion);
- a counter;
- a display for showing the measurement results.

One of the two measurement signals e_1 and e_2 and an appropriately phase-shifted reference voltage are brought to the inputs of the multiplier.

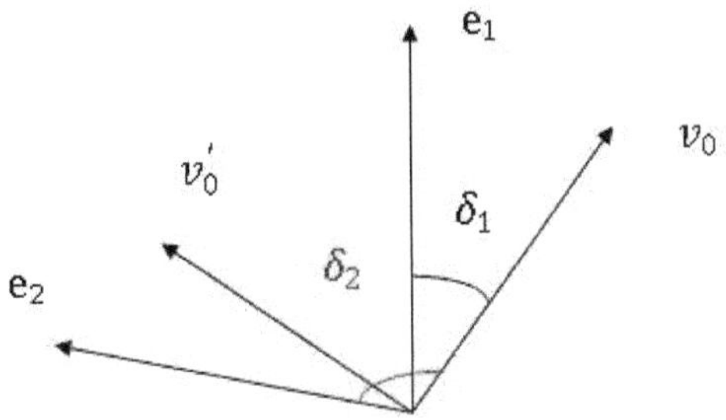

FIGURE 1.3
Phasor diagram of the voltages.

With reference to Fig. 1.3, the reference signal $v_o(\mathrm{t})$, assumed with 0° phase shift, is sent to the multiplier, in order to be converted by the double-ramp converter. The first two measured values are obtained:

$$\frac{1}{T}\int_T e_1(t)v_0(t)dt = E_1V_o cos(\delta_1) \tag{1.1}$$

$$\frac{1}{T}\int_T e_2(t)v_0(t)dt = E_2V_o cos(\delta_2) \tag{1.2}$$

where T is the measuring interval, E_1 and and V_o the root mean square of the voltage drop e_1 and v_0, respectively, and δ the phase difference. Then, by imposing to this signal a phase shift of 90°, the following values are obtained:

$$\frac{1}{T}\int_T e_1(t)v_0^{'}(t)dt = E_1V_o cos(90-\delta_1) = E_1V_0 sin(\delta_1) \tag{1.3}$$

$$\frac{1}{T}\int_T e_2(t)v_0^{'}(t)dt = E_2V_o cos(\delta_2-90) = E_2V_0 sin(\delta_2) \tag{1.4}$$

The instrument processing unit is now able to evaluate the phase shift between e_1 and e_2 as:

$$\angle\epsilon = arctg\left(\frac{E_2V_0 sin(\delta_2)}{E_2V_o cos(\delta_2)}\right) - arctg\left(\frac{E_1V_0 sin(\delta_1)}{E_1V_o cos(\delta_1)}.\right) \tag{1.5}$$

The magnitude of the unknown impedance is:

$$|Z_x| = R_s\frac{E_1}{E_2}. \tag{1.6}$$

From these values the phase and quadrature component of the unknown impedance are then calculated.

From the above equations, it is clear that the method is affected by high uncertainty for low impedance. The instrument solves this problem by carrying out two other measurements with a voltage v_0 out of phase by 180°.

The circuit of Fig. 1.2 has the drawback of implementing the crucial part of the measurement algorithm, related to the projection of the voltage and current phasors on the axes (multiplier and phase shifter circuit) by means of analog circuitry, affected by high uncertainty.

A solution to this problem involves the immediate digital conversion of the two waveforms e_1 and e_2 (Fig. 1.4). The knowledge of the two digitized waveforms allows to directly realize the numerical measurement algorithm, by measuring the ratio between the effective values and the initial phase difference, and by estimating the zero crossing of the two waveforms. In the ideal case, two samples with the same index i of the arrays of the two waveforms, acquired at the sampling rate f_c, are out of phase by $1/f_c$, due to the switching in the multiplexer. Therefore, the systematic component of this phase error is corrected by correcting the power factor correction through an index. A simple implementation consists in applying a sine fitting algorithm to each waveform and, once the models have been identified, proceed analytically to determine the impedance. For example, in this way, in a polar representation of the impedance, the effective values and the phase difference can be estimated numerically.

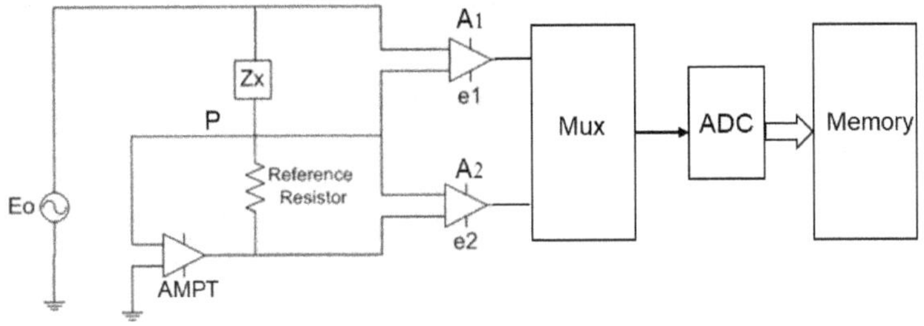

FIGURE 1.4
Architecture of an impedance meter with immediate numerical conversion.

1.2 Bioimpedance Measurements in Aesthetics Medicine

Biompedance spectroscopy is considered as a powerful method, painless and harmless, for characterizing the biophysical features of the tissues. By and large, the measurement of the biological impedance requires the injection of an electrical current, crossing the biological tissue under test. Naturally, no damage or disturbance of any kind should happen to that tissue. From a physiological point of view, it means that no excitable tissue should be stimulated (such as nerve or muscle, especially skeletal, cardiac, or smooth).

The bioimpedance depends on the applied signal frequency and amplitude, and it varies significantly according to the type of tissue, namely its structure, composition, and health status. The electrical properties of biological tissues are related to the microscopic structure of cellular media and, at macroscopic level, to the physiologic and pathological state of organs. Thus, the bioimpedance varies from tissue to tissue and subject to subject. Moreover, most tissues are anisotropic, thus, impedance varies according to the measurement direction.

Impedance measurements methods can contribute to successfully investigate the physiological or pathological status of biological tissues. In particular, skin impedance measurement and analysis could be applied in the fields of cosmetology, dermatological research, and so on.

In a narrow way, skin impedance is the response of a specific skin region to an externally applied electrical field. Electrical current has been used in medicine for more than a century. For example, the biostimulation, such as cardioversion of atrial fibrillation, uses low-frequency or direct current, which causes spasms of the muscles [14]. High-frequency current in the range of 0.3 Hz to 10.0 MHz, or radiofrequency (RF) current, produces thermal effects on biological tissue that is reliant on its electrical properties.

In aesthetic medicine, the use of RF, as an energy source for selective electro-thermolysis, is a rather new approach [15]. Systems that integrate the RF current have been in development for several years, but they become popular only recently. Studies using these new technologies are employed in hair removal, skin rejuvenation, and wrinkle reduction. The RF thermal effects promote skin tightening by immediate collagen contraction and delayed collagen remodelling process [16].

The effects of first-generation monopolar and bipolar RF devices are often partial or even unpredictable, probably due to the differences in individual skin impedance, uncounted during the treatments. Indeed, the bioimpedance is known to vary between different individuals (according to gender, race, age, and so on), as well as in the same patients between different body areas, and current skin humidity. Moreover, bioimpedance changes due to the topical administration of moisturizing agents or local anaesthesia [17]. Thus, natural or induced alteration of the individual skin impedance may have an effect on the uniform delivery of the effective energy conveyed into the tissue by the RF systems. Therefore, a real-time personalized energy delivery, according to skin impedance, allows a remarkable proper and safer non-ablative skin tightening with more consistent and predictable results.

During non-ablative RF skin tightening and body contouring, the RF energy is conveyed into the skin. In order to grant a constant and consistent energy delivery, the power delivered needs to be normalized to the skin impedance. Therefore, monitoring the skin impedance in real time turns out to be crucial. Usually, before each pulse, the operator measures the bioimpedance and sets the device. Some devices measure the impedance between the handpiece contact pointed on the surface of the skin and a second plate attached to the back of the patient, by taking into account the full-body capacitive impedance. Other treatments, using at least a bipolar device (Aurora; Syneron, Yokneam Illit, Israel), exploit two electrodes on the surface of the skin (resistive impedance). Meanwhile, the EndyMed PRO (EndyMed) measures in real time the impedance, and allows a customization of the delivered energy according to differences in skin impedance [18–20].

Bioimpedance has been used to study the skin hydration level and the moisturizing effect of sericin (a silk protein akin to the natural moisturizing factor), and it is widely used in skin cosmetics [21].

Healthy skin is perceived as a clean, soft, flexible, moist, and nearly without wrinkles tissue. The water content determines the skin smoothness and softness, acting especially on the outer layer of the epidermis. When water content decreases, keratin becomes progressively less flexible, and so the skin becomes less soft and flexible, resulting in an acceleration of the aging process [22]. Hydration measurement is useful to assess the function of anti-aging and miniaturization treatments in cosmetology [23–25]. In addition, skin hydration monitoring is a consolidate and valuable technique in dermatology to investigate various diseases and evaluate the effectiveness of medical treatments [24]. For example, the electrical conductance and transepidermal water loss may be useful for monitoring the primary effect of the therapy and for the final evaluation of healing of patients undergoing treatments of chronic scaly hand eczema [26].

Skin impedance is an important aspect of bioimpedance and can be used to analyze the condition of the human body. Accurate researches have been carried out on a combination of skin characteristics and bioimpedance parameters [27, 28].

In order to clearly expose the model of skin impedance, it is indispensable to figure out the anatomy of skin. The development of any biomedical device or measurement technique cannot neglect a deep knowledge of the physiological and chemical structure of the skin. The skin is the most extensive organ of the human body, with an average surface area, in adults, of almost 2 m^2. The skin is extremely dynamic, due to its ability to absorb mechanical stress, prevent excessive loss of liquids, facilitate heat exchange, protect from sun radiation, and so on. Such a wide variety of functions are ensured by three superimposed layers of different chemical composition and morphological structure (Fig. 1.5): the *dermis*, the *viableepidermis* and the *stratuscorneum*.

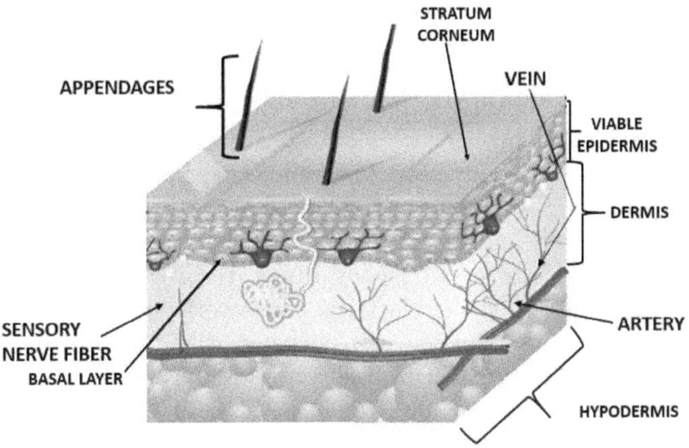

FIGURE 1.5
Schematic representation of human skin and its main components.

The deepest part of the skin is the *dermis* (or corium), which nourishes and supports the epidermis, with thickness varying from about 500–2000 μm according to the body site [29]. It contains a connective tissue, formed from an interwoven network of collagen and elastic fibers. The dermis contains numerous blood and lymph vessels, nerves, nerve endings, and sweat glands, providing the transpiration and the base of the pilosebaceous system. In transdermal drug delivery applications, drugs are supposed to be preliminary carried into the dermis and then into blood vessels.

The next layer is called *viableepidermis*, with thickness also greatly variable, around 150 μm. It is divided into four sublayers vertically: stratum lucidum, stratum granulosum, stratum spinosum, and stratum basale [30]. The viable epidermis is hydrophilic, since it is composed by 40 % of protein, around 40 %–60 % of water and lipid and besides there are no blood vessels [31].

The *stratum corneum* is the most superficial layer of the skin. It consists of flat cells and corneocytes, which are dead cells without nuclei, embedded into a highly-ordered and dense lipid matrix, which form an impermeable lining and a natural barrier in transdermal transport [32, 33]. This barrier allows the retention of water inside the body and guarantees protection from external substances, such as toxins and microorganisms. The thickness of stratum corneum varies considerably among different individuals and different body sites. As an example, the thickness of the forearm is about 10–40 μm [34]. Moreover, it has been proven that the stratum corneum has a negative charge [35, 36], which promotes the transport through the skin of cations rather than anions. Additionally, the skin has a pH between 3 and 4 [33, 37]. Therefore, some techniques such as mesoporation and iontophoresis, which exploit both the negative charge and the pH of the skin, can be used in order to increase its permeability. In brief, the stratum corneum properties highly affect the measurement of skin impedance and the assessment of skin permeability due to its peculiar physiological structure.

One of the most promising techniques for the characterization of the physiological and structural properties of biological tissues is based on the evaluation of the electrical conduction phenomena within them. In particular, Electrical Impedance Spectroscopy (EIS) measurements [38,39] are in fact absolutely non-destructive and low invasive. Basically, EIS applies low-intensity electric currents, over a wide frequency range, to provide more meaningful independent information on the electrical characteristics of a tissue. In general, electrical models of the tissues are developed and identified using EIS. In EIS experiments, the perturbation is constituted by a sinusoidal signal of slight amplitude, from tens to hundreds of mV [40] of a sinewave $\Delta Esen(\omega t)$ superimposed on a continuous bias voltage, E_0. The system response to this perturbation is confidently a sinusoidal current: $\Delta Isen(\omega t\text{-}\phi)$. To obtain a linear response of the tissue, a sufficiently small amplitude of the applied signal is chosen. By varying the frequency of the applied voltage, the impedance of the material under examination is obtained as a function of the frequency. The spectrum of this impedance is typically represented graphically by means of the Bode and Nyquist diagrams.

In this type of experimental investigation, two main sources of uncertainty are highlighted: the electrode polarization and the inductance of the conductor cables. They occur at different frequency intervals: for low frequency (<100 Hz), the burden of the electrode polarization is dominant, while for high frequency (>1 MHz), the inductance of the cable involves significant uncertainty. However, suitable mathematical models to correct the deterministic part can be defined, starting from the actual measurements data. These models return a set of values for the parameters under consideration, used to derive an equivalent circuit model as close as possible to the reality. Obviously, there are some peculiarities of the electrical properties of biological tissues. Firstly, in biological tissues, the charge carriers of electric currents are represented by ions. For this reason, the conductivity of biological tissues is strongly dependent on parameters such as concentration, effective charge, diffusion coefficients and the types of ions involved in the process. In electrical circuits, the current density does not affect the properties of the circuit (at least up to about 100 A/cm^2) and passive circuits follow the Ohm's law. On the other hand, the linearity of the tissues properties is considered as constant until the injected current does not exceed 1 mA/cm^2 (this value is also a function of the frequency). Therefore, the need to identify a linearity region is evident.

Although the properties of electronic circuits and biological tissues are different, the latter can be described by means of suitable circuit models. The experimental results of the impedance spectroscopy of a tissue can be analyzed in terms of an equivalent electrical circuit model [28, 41], in order to find the impedance equals or that reflects to the measured data. The type of electrical components of the model and their interconnections control the shape of the impedance spectrum of the model. In an electrical model, each component represents a physical process of conduction within and on the surface of the biological tissue. The choice of the model derives from the knowledge of its characteristics. The same impedance spectrum can be modelled by multiple equivalent electrical circuits, so the model must be selected correctly before its use.

The impedance of a biological tissue can be measured starting from an interaction between an electric current with the tissue at cellular and molecular level. The electrical properties of skin have been studied for over a century. An equivalent circuit, with a resistor (R_e) in series with the parallel of a resistor (R_{skin}) and a particualr capacitor (CPE), has been used successfully to describe the skin's electrical properties (Fig. 1.6). In this model, CPE

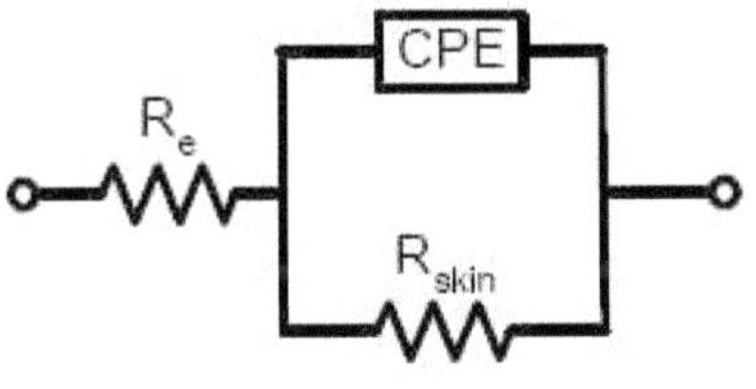

FIGURE 1.6
Equivalent circuit of human skin impedance measurement.

is a pseudo-capacitance, represented by a special element, called Constant Phase Element (CPE), as described by Cole-Cole [42]. It represents the properties of the stratum corneum, the skin's most superficial layer. Conversely, R_e represents the resistance associated with the deeper tissues. From this circuit, more complex linear and nonlinear circuits have been proposed in order to model skin's electrical properties more closely. Additional resistors and capacitors, as well as inductors, voltage sources, and diodes, have ben involved. Nevertheless, the abovementioned circuit has proved to be an optimal linear model, where additional resistors and capacitors do not provide statistically significant improvement.

A better understanding of the impedance characteristics of the skin, as well as the optimization of the skin impedance models, are imperative in order to optimize the evaluation of the tissue health status.

The tissue health varies in relation to physiological and pathological variations, and, similarly, bioimpedance varies from an healthy to a diseased tissue. As a matter of fact, cancerous and sane tissues differ morphologically; thus, it can be assumed that these differences induce a change in electrical proprieties. Indeed, the impedance of a normal tissue is higher, since the cancerous tissue needs more blood to continue its fast and uncontrolled growth. In fact, the blood is a good conductor of electricity and the cancerous tissue has a lot of blood; this latter shows a less impedance path to the electrical current. The literature reports many studies about the difference in impedance measurements between cancerous and normal tissues [43].

Bioimpedance analysis is a practical and reliable method for the early diagnosis of lymphedema in patients under treatment for breast cancer [44]. Electrical impedance spectra have been successfully used to distinguish between malignant melanoma and benign skin lesions [45]. Among the studies relative to pathological tissues, the most promising areas seem to be, on one hand, the characterization of cancerous tissues, and, on the other hand, the study of ischemia during organ conservation and transplantation. The assessment of tissue perfusion/ischemia levels is particularly crucial for preoperative monitoring of transplanted heart and liver, or for postoperative monitoring of transplanted muscle flaps, and in plastic and reconstructive surgery. It is expected that in-depth analysis will be provided by further studies on these topics.

1.2.1 Total Body Bioimpedance

Impedance techniques are exploited to assess changes in orientation, volume, or distribution of tissue fluids, connected to physiological activity.

Numerous studies have proven the usefulness of bioelectrical impedance analysis (BIA) for assessing body composition [46]. This method strength relies on its scarce invasiveness, high portability, safety, fast and easy execution, as well as on its low cost. Therefore, BIA presents many characteristics of an ideal technique for studying body composition [47].

BIA is based on the evidence of a frequency-dependent impedance of the body tissues to a low-frequency alternating current (generally sinusoidal). The impedance (Z) of an isotropic conductor (i.e., a cylinder) is proportional to its length (L), and inversely proportional to its cross–sectional area (A). Consequently, at a specific frequency, the electric volume of a generic conductive material can be assessed by its length and impedance. However, when the conducting material can be assumed to behave as a pure resistor $Z = R$, and thus the following formula is valid for the volume $V = \rho\ L^2/R$: $R = \rho\ L/A = \rho\ L^2/V$, , where ρ is the resistivity of the conducting material and V equals AL. The factor L^2/R is called impedance index.

Clearly, the human body is not a homogeneous isotropic cylinder, and it has neither a uniform cross-sectional area, nor can be described by a single cylinder, but at least by five cylinders (two arms, two legs, and the trunk). Moreover, body composition is extremely varying and cannot be crossed by a uniform current. By taking clearly into account such limitations, the human body can be approximated to a cylinder, whose length represents the height, since it is easier to measure the height than the conductive length, which is usually from wrist to ankle.

Finally, an empirical relationship can be established between the impedance quotient ($Length^2/R$) and the volume of water, which contains electrolytes carrying the electrical current through the body. The relationship has a proper coefficient, which depends on different factors, and takes into account the actual geometry of the body and the body's segments anatomy [48]. Consequently, errors can arise from the variations of body segments, shapes, the ratio height to conductive length, and changes in conductive material resistivity.

Bioimpedance is a complex parameter which combines a resistance (R, Ω), arising from extra- and intracellular fluid, and a reactance (Xc, Ω), linked to the capacitance of cells membranes [49, 50].

Quite a few instruments are available to measure impedance for a wide range of frequency (from 1 kHz to 1 MHz). Most single-frequency BIA analyzers operate at 50 kHz. Therefore, it is advisable to limit the impedance measurement to a smaller frequency range. By and large, at high frequency (>50 kHz), the current crosses the cell membranes, and it is associated with both intra and extracellular fluid. On the other hand, at very-low frequency, the current passes through the extracellular fluid because it cannot cross the cellular membrane, which acts as an insulator.

In any case, BIA measures the electrical properties of body tissues and represents a valuable technique for assessing body composition parameters, such as the Total Body Water (TBW) [50]. TBW includes Intracellular Water (ICW) and Extracellular Water (ECW). ICW is found within the cells and tissues, and determines cell and tissue volumes. The ECW is composed of blood, lymph, and so on [51].

In epidemiology and clinical practice, the body composition is assessed by means of the bicompartimental model. It merely divides the body into Fat Mass (FM) and Fat-Free mass (FFM). FFM, also known as lean body mass or muscle mass, under physiological conditions, includes the non-fat components of the human body, such as skeletal muscle, internal organs and visceral proteins ($\approx$ 20 %), bones with bone mineral content ($\approx$ 7 %), as well as extracellular ($\approx$ 29 %) and intracellular water ($\approx$ 44 %). Whereas, FM indicates the water-free body component [52, 53].

The schematic representation of the body composition is shown in Fig. 1.7: it includes fat-free mass (FFM), total body water (TBW), intracellular water (ICW), extracellular water (ECW), and body cell mass (BCM).

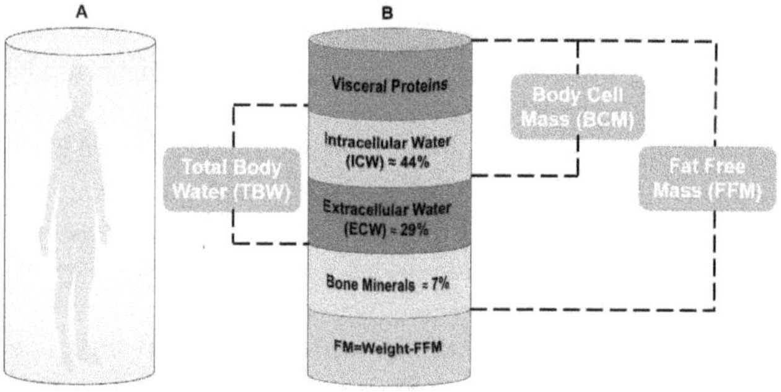

FIGURE 1.7
Human body representation in BIA as: (A) a conducting cylinder and (B) the composition schematic model.

In the clinical practice, BIA is assessed by means of a body composition analyzer, an instrument which injects a constant current and measures the electrical impedance of the body (Z_B) by a standard four-electrodes configuration. In single-frequency BIA, a low- and constant-amplitude ($\leq$1 mA) alternating current, generally at 50 kHz, crosses the surface electrodes placed on hand and foot. The current is injected through two current electrodes, while two voltage electrodes measure the corresponding potential drop. Other BIA devices use a different electrode configuration, such as foot-to-foot, or hand-to-hand electrodes (Bipedal BIA) [54].

Single-frequency BIA at 50 kHz permits to estimate FFM and TBW, but not differences in ICW. Moreover, single-frequency BIA can be used in normal or not so much altered condition, since its outcomes are based on empirical equations and theories obtained by healthy subjects.

BIA can operate using electrical current at different frequency bandwidths (multi-frequency BIA), ranging from low (1 kHz) to high (500 kHz) frequency. This allows to measure the BW, FFM, FM, ICW, and ECW compartments by using empirical linear regression models. Patel et al., [55] agree that for critical subjects, single-frequency-BIA is more accurate to asses TBW; while, in general, multi-frequency BIA is more accurate to predict ECW. Even if, according to Olde-Rikkert et al., [56], multi-frequency BIA cannot reveal changes in distribution or movement of fluid between extracellular and intracellular spaces in elderly people.

The measurement of bioelectrical impedance is influenced by numerous factors and its standardization is essential for a fruitful use of the method [57]. Main uncertainty sources are related to instrumentation, operator, environment, and the subject under test. The intra-instrumental repeatability

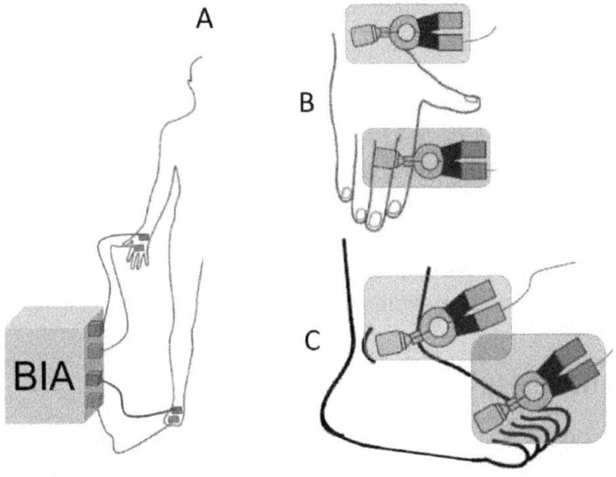

FIGURE 1.8
Typical electrode configurations for human body bioimpedance measurement (A). Red electrodes inject current while blue electrodes measure voltage placed on right hand (B) and right foot (C).

can be determined through repeated measurements of circuits with a known impedance (or resistance). It is absolutely essential to check the accuracy of an impedance meter before and during its use in epidemiological studies and after long periods of inactivity. Moreover, it is important that the electrodes are adequately placed and the connection cables are properly shielded and connected straight without coming into contact with each other on a non-conductive surface [58].

During a BIA procedure, which lasts about 5 minutes, an operator attaches the electrodes on the patients body. The patient can be in lying or standing condition: the posture is crucial for the interpretation of the impedance data. The patient should not apply moisturises on hands or foot, since they can artificially modify the electrical conductivity of the skin. In general, it is advisable to avoid food or drink caffeine for 4 hours before the exam, because the stomach contents can interfere with impedance measurement. Furthermore, in the post-absorptive phase, the passage of liquids into the circulation stream can produce excessive uncertainty [59]. In addition, patients should not neither workout 12 hours before, nor wear metal jewellery during the exam [58].

Another factor to take into account is the ambient temperature. In theory, it is able to influence the impedance measurement through its effects on the skin microcirculation and on the hydro-electrolytic homeostasis. In fact, the skin microcirculation is able to dilate in response to an increase in the skin temperature. On the contrary, the reduction of skin temperature produces vasoconstriction, with a decrease in the hematic flow. This explains why higher impedance values can be recorded after skin cooling [60]. In the presence of fever, the BIA is unreliable, since it records artificially low impedance values.

Nowadays several more accurate methods to measure body composition are available, such as densitometry (underwater weighing), hydrometry (deuterium dilution), Echo-MRI, and total body potassium counting [61, 62]. In spite of that, these methods present complex measurement protocols and require specialized expertise and costly equipment, limiting their application in clinical settings. Therefore, despite of the aforementioned limitations, BIA represents a noninvasive, portable, low-cost, and reliable method for assessing body composition in both clinical and non-clinical settings.

1.2.2 Localized Bioimpedance

Body composition assessment is considered as a key factor for the evaluation of general health status of humans. In clinical practice, measurement of total body bioimpedance is the most broadly used method for quickly estimating whole body compartments, in terms of total-body water, fat-free mass, fat mass, or other body compartments.

In order to overcome the limitation of the whole-body BIA technique, where large changes in a body district are only partially indicated by the total body impedance, a segment-localized bioimpedance analysis is used. Segmental BIA is mainly applied to assess the composition of the limbs, by detecting the balance and distribution of lean mass, as well as any asymmetries. All above, it is a more precise technique than whole-body BIA, since, unlike the latter which considers the human body as a single cylinder, segmental BIA approximates the body to a set of five cylinders (two arms, two legs, and the trunk). Our body, in fact, is not a homogeneous conductor: each segment has its own particular electrical and geometric characteristics. Additionally, the impedance of the limbs is considerably greater than the trunk one, due to the smaller section of these latter and the more uniform distribution of the tissues inside them, with the absence of cavity. Moreover, segmental BIA achieves a better estimation of Fat Free Mass (FFM), indeed it detects the fluctuation in extra-cellular fluid (ECF) due to differences in posture. Furthermore, it is more precise than the ankle-foot method, and, by giving a better estimation of TBW, than whole-body BIA [63, 64].

The BIA is a powerful method to determine human health condition, in addition, its application is useful in disease diagnoses. Since, fluctuations like fat-free mass, fat mass and total body water from normal limits are parameters used in several studies to evaluate and analyze the changes in disorders of different kind of diseases. Therefore, it is useful to analyze the impedance response in limited areas, as an example, portion of tissues in melanoma studies. By referring to the limb, BIA can investigate the upper limbs edema post mastectomy, or study of panniculopathies of the lower limbs before and after treatment; about the abdomen, BIA studies the gastric empting study, visceral fat study.

Recent applications of localized BIA include neuromuscular disease diagnosis. According to the anatomical characteristic of muscles fibres, once applied the electrical current to the muscle, the detected impedance decreases along the direction parallel to the muscle fiber, while increases when the electrical current cross transversely the muscle. These observations are useful to determinate the effective resistivity, which reflects the neuromuscular function and status [65].

Different studies have also addressed the possibility to apply BIA in Sport Medicine to evaluate physical performance and assess athletes muscle strength and sport performance [66, 67].

More in general, BIA is a useful tool in clinical practice, as it allows to evaluate the biological fluid amount. In particular, the alteration in the patients' hydration by pathological condition such as hemodialysis [68] or ambulatory peritoneal dialysis [69], and liver cirrhosis [70] can be assessed.

Another well-established approach, which includes impedance of extremities, is limb Impedance Plethysmography (IPG), that has found a remarkable place in clinical practice. IPG measures variation in the electrical impedance corresponding to a change in the blood volume of a specific body segments, say chest, calf, or any other regions of the body. In particular, IPG can be used to measure blood flow in a limb or digit; hence, this technique has been widely applied for the evaluation of patients at risk or suspected to have lower extremity Deep Venous Thrombosis (DVT) [71]. An example of its application requires the placement of two electrodes together with a blood pressure cuff, placed around the thigh. The blood volume can be manipulated by inflation of the pneumatic cuff around the thigh, because this latter is inversely proportional to the electrical impedance. Once obstructed the blood flow out of the calf, the rate of impedance variation can recognize the obstruction. The blood, compared to the tissues, can be considered as a good electrical conductor; every changes in the conductibility of body region produces an electrical impedance variation proportional to the electrical currents that flows in that specific body region. Therefore, a decrease in electrical impedance denotes the introduction of a certain amount blood in the area of interest.

In brief, IPG is easy to perform and turns out to be non-invasive compared to venography; it does not require skilled operator and can help physician to detect alteration in blood flow, DVT, arterial and veins insufficiency or occlusive disease, blood clots in limbs or pulmonary emboli [72, 73].

Cardiovascular monitoring is generally performed using invasive techniques that give very precise information. IPG represents an alternative that allows the study of the cardiovascular system in a totally non-invasive and risk-free way for patients. It can be used above all to measure the variation of a quantity rather than its absolute value, the impedance variation of a section of the chest due meanly to breathing but also to cardiac activity. In general, Plethysmography concerns the change in volume of a body tissue.

Another application which exploits the characteristic impedance of the tissue and blood in the thorax, which changes with respiration and the cardiac cycle largely because of the changes in thoracic vascular volume, is Thoracic Electrical Bioimpedance (TEB), also known as Impedance Cardiography (ICG). The ICG is essentially similar to the IPG procedure: one pair of electrodes, usually placed at the base of the neck, injects an alternating electric current (frequency range of 20 Hz to 100 kHz). Correspondingly, another two electrodes, placed on xiphoid or xiphisternal joint, measure the related voltage. TEB depends on biological composition, breathings, and by the blood circulation and blood volume of thoracic vessels. After processing to remove the respiratory component, the change in impedance from the baseline impedance, Z_0, is related to the cardiac cycle. Therefore, the analysis of Z_0 allows to evaluate the heart health status along with calculations of certain hemodynamic parameters including stroke volume, cardiac output, cardiac index, systemic vascular resistance, and left work index [58, 74].

As earlier mentioned, BIA analysis seems to be a handy and reliable technique for early diagnosing lymphedema, especially for the follow-up of patients under treatment for cancer [44]. Within this framework, the characterization of cancerous tissues in an important application of bioimpedance spectrometry. It is well known that cancerous tissue presents a different morphology compared to healthy tissue, and this different can be linked to changes in the electrical properties.

In fact, EIS can be used to detect skin lesion and malignant melanomas, since it has been proved that EIS is affected by histologically visible skin alterations which is correlate to histologic diagnosis [75]. Therefore, EIS represents a diagnostic decision support technique for malignant melanoma diagnosis [45].

In conclusion, the applications of BIA in the different clinic fields are innumerable and full of potential, although further research/studies are necessary, especially in the heads of aesthetic medicine, diabetes, and orthopaedics. In the following chapters, an innovative application of the EIS for aesthetic treatments will be shown.

1.3 Biompedance Measurements in Diabetology

Diabetes is one of the most spread non-communicable diseases worldwide. Globally, the number of people with diabetes, according to International Diabetes Federation, is currently around 463 million and is expected to increase to 700 million by 2045. This disease is the fifth leading cause of death in most developed countries; after all, four million deaths are related to diabetes and its complications [76]. Diabetes treatment and related complications costs affect health services and national productivity, as well as individuals and families. Its financial burden has a relevant impact on the economy of the society.

Strictly speaking, diabetes is a condition that impairs the body's ability to process blood glucose, otherwise informally known as "blood sugar".

Blood glucose is one of the main energy source of our body and it derives principally from food intake. The hormone, which promotes the absorption of glucose from the blood into cells to be used for energy, is the insulin produced by the islets of Langerhans of the pancreas. When our body does not produce insulin, or its amount is not sufficient, the glucose is not able to reach the cells, and over time, its accumulation in blood can cause serious health problems.

Different kinds of diabetes can occur, and managing the condition depends on the type. Not all diabetes forms arise from obesity or unhealthy lifestyle, but appear also in childhood indeed. Although there is no permanent cure, diabetes can be managed and patients can stay healthy. The most common types of are type 1, type 2, and gestational diabetes. Among them, people with type-1 diabetes are insulin-dependent: they must take artificial insulin daily to stay alive, since their body fails to produce it. Therefore, the frequent monitoring of blood glucose concentration is a crucial part of diabetic management. Nowadays, insulin treatment strategies consist of either multiple-daily insulin injections or continuous subcutaneous insulin infusion with a pump.

Patients with chronic conditions, such as diabetes mellitus, require self-management in homecare settings; in fact, the self-monitoring of blood glucose (SMBG) (by the patient themselves or with the assistance of relatives), in daily life, is made by a blood strip and a lancing device (Fig. 1.9). Although devices tend to be almost fully automated and require only a few simple user operations to go from sample preparation to test result, frequent finger pricks can become rather painful if a regular monitoring is necessary [77].

Despite modern devices (smaller, more reliable, with reduced blood sample requirement, faster) and easier to use compared to those used about 15 years ago, there is an increasing demand for non-invasive analytical methods to achieve effective glucose monitoring in diabetics. A painless device would motivate people suffering from diabetes to monitor their glucose concentration more frequently or even continuously.

The progress of the Blood Glucose Monitoring Devices (BGMD) is more oriented to non-invasive method, in order to avoid blood drawing, the insertion of needles, or any kind of sensor under the skin. The main aim is to measure blood glucose level only placing the sensor on the human target area. In view of the fact that minimally invasive devices, continuously monitoring blood glucose, are already available. However, these devices use subcutaneous sensors, and they are not really comfortable for patients. Moreover, they require continuous calibration and have to be removed and placed surgically by a physician.

The most popular blood glucose monitors almost exclusively adopt enzymatic analysis methods, based on glucose oxidase and glucose dehydrogenase, owing to their better sensitivity, reproducibility, and easy maintenance, as well as their affordable cost [78]. The enzymatic reaction products are detected photometrically or electrochemically in glucose test strips and glucometers.

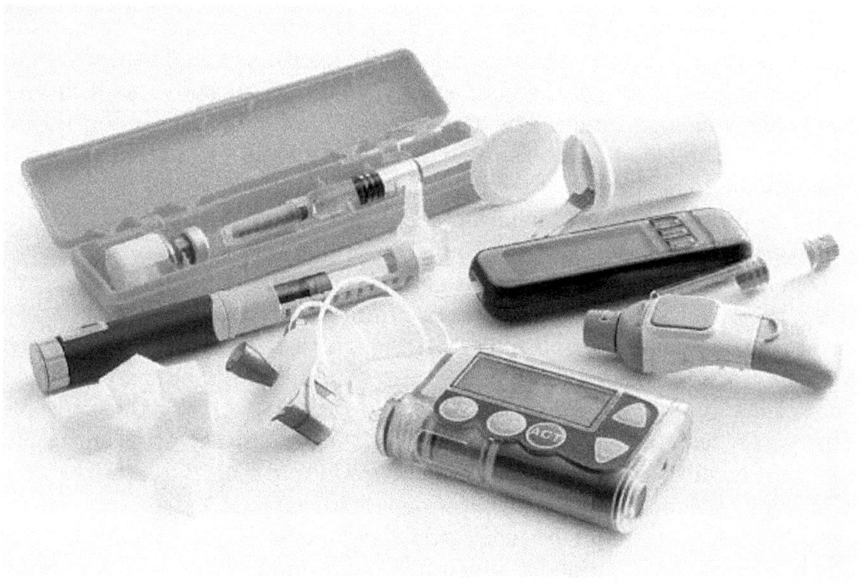

FIGURE 1.9
Different insulin sets: syringe with a vial of insulin, glucometer with test strips, lancing device, infusion set, sugar lumps, and insulin pen.

In the reflectometric method, the intensity of the colour of the chromogen, generated by the reaction, is measured. On the other hand, the impedancemetric method measures the electrical conductivity of the blood, induced by the current generated by the redox reaction itself. An example of a typical glucometer is shown in Fig. 1.10).

A fist classification of non-invasive blood glucose monitoring (NBGM) could be based on their technologies. Optical monitoring technologies involving infrared (IR), mid-infrared (MIR) spectroscopy based on light in the 2500 nm to 10000 nm spectrum and near-infrared (NIR) region of the electromagnetic spectrum (750 to 2500 nm), are available for glucose detection. Once a tissue is illuminated, the light attenuation and its resulting spectrum, which represent its optical signature, are strongly related to physicochemical parameters such as tissue composition, changes in body temperature, blood pressure, skin hydration, concentrations of triglyceride, and albumin [79].

However, it is difficult to figure out glucose-specific information from such spectra. Especially because glucose molecules are predominantly located in the interstitial fluid, at the junction between epidermis and dermis; rather than in dermis, which is the target region for spectroscopy [80]. In addition, the interstitial glucose concentration is proportional to the blood concentration, albeit with a delay of 10 min [81]. NIR and MIR spectroscopy are applied on the earlobe, finger pulp forearm, lip mucosa, oral mucosa, tongue, nasal

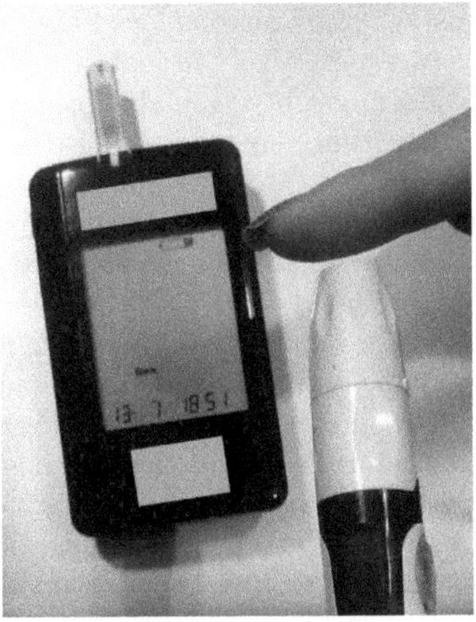

FIGURE 1.10
Glucometer with test strip and pen blood lancet. A small drop of blood, gained by pricking the finger with a lancet, is placed on a disposable test strip and than analyzed by the device which calculates the blood glucose level. The meter finally displays the level in units of mg/dL or mmol/L.

septum, cheek, and arm. The measurement takes approximately 1 min and allows for quasi-continuous glucose monitoring for one day without recalibration [82]. NIR diffuse reflectance measurements, performed on the finger, show a correlation with blood glucose; nevertheless, the predictions are often not sufficiently accurate to be clinically acceptable [83].

Another method based on the assessment of the glucose concentration of interstitial fluid (ISF), as abovementioned closely related to the blood glucose level, has been applied to continuous glucose monitoring using impedance measurements [84]. In particular, the measurement of normal skin impedance has been proposed to determine the volume of the ISF extracted transdermally, which is linked in turn to glucose concentration. Actually, transdermal permeation rate of glucose molecules is inversely proportional to the skin impedance in the normal direction. Furthermore, transdermal permeation of the skin defines the volume of extracted ISF.

Impedance spectroscopy has been proposed as possible approach for non-invasive glycaemia monitoring. However only few studies report data about impedance related to glucose concentration, especially below the MHz band [85]. Li et al. investigate the dielectric properties of aqueous solutions with different glucose concentrations, by considering also the blood volume pulsation in a full cardiac cycle, and by measuring bioimpedance difference for NBGM [86].

Tissue dielectric constant has been employed also as an indicator of skin water content, whose changes, especially in foot, are linked to diabetes mellitus. The dielectric constant might be a valuable technique to screen for early changes in foot skin features, that may tend to cause diabetes mellitus-related edema [87].

Another study suggests that tissue dielectric constant, used to assess skin water content, is inversely related to the glycated haemoglobin, HbA1c. Changes in dermal water is related to glucose control as measured by HbA1c or fasting glucose. The HbA1c value reveals the average plasma glucose levels during the last 2 to 3 months and has been considered, for a long time, the standard for assessing blood glucose control over longer periods [88].

The electrical impedance measurement of blood has a positive correlation with blood glucose values. Impedance sensing devices, with different working electrode areas, can investigate the glucose concentrations present in the human blood. Within this framework, the impedance value increases with the rise of glucose concentration in blood, independently from the specific body area under test [89].

Finally, it is beyond doubt that despite of the promising advances, we are only at the beginning of non-invasive glucose biosensor development, which combines accurate real-time glucose monitoring, with long-term stability and appreciable accuracy.

1.3.1 Glycemic Crisis Detection

Diabetes Mellitus is a chronic metabolic disorder characterized by endogenous inability to control glycaemic excursions. Injecting exogenous insulin to restore normoglycaemia is not only a life-safing treatment for type-1 diabetes mellitus patients, but also a benefit for the patients with type-2 diabetes mellitus that cannot properly clear circulating blood glucose, owing to insulin resistance. Sustained periods of hyper- or hypo-glycaemia, characterized by oscillations between these states, can adversely affect health status. In fact, a poor glycaemic control leads to long-term complications, including retinopathy, nephropathy, neuropathy, an increased risk of cardiovascular disease, and so, a significant increase in mortality.

Hyperglycemia refers to a condition with an excessive amount of glucose circulating in the blood plasma; therefore, it develops in conditions with a low net insulin actions. The symptoms of hyperglycemia include: high glucose levels ($>$ 200 mg glucose/dL) in blood and urine, frequent urination, and increased thirst. Indeed, hyperglycemia induces platelet hyper-reactivity, which increases thrombosis, cardiac cell death, reduces coronary collateral blood flow, and also leads to endothelial cell dysfunction [90].

On the other hand, hypoglycemia, which literally means low blood glucose concentration, is a very common secondary effect to insulin therapy in diabetics. Its diagnosis requires glucose level $<$ 2.5–2.8 mmol/l or equivalently ($<$ 45–50 mg/dl) for men and $<$ 1.9–2.2 mmol/l ($<$ 35–40 mg/dl) for women.

Its typical symptoms include: sweating, tachycardia, tremors, anxiety, dizziness, visual changes confusion, and even convulsions. In most cases, glucose level falls only slightly below normal and it is easily treated by consuming foods that quickly raise plasma glucose levels, such as pure sugar, or fruit juice and candy. However, severe diabetic hypoglycemia can lead to hospitalization [91]. Glycaemic control remains the major intervention for prevention and the correction of both hyperglycemia and hypoglycemia.

Remembering that, diabetes is diagnosed if there are its typical symptoms (polyuria, polydipsia, unexplained weight loss) and a random glucose level > 200 mg/dl. A fasting glucose of > 126 mg/dl or a glucose of > 200 mg/dl 2 hours after a 75-g glucose load, are also diagnostic [92]. However, determining the optimal insulin dosing is not easy. It depends on several factors such as: age, weight, pubertal stage, duration and stage of diabetes, injection site, food intake and meal distribution, physical activity, nominal insulin sensitivity, blood glucose results (and glycosylated hemoglobin), and undercurrent illnesses.

Mathematical modelling of physiological systems is widely applied in all the science fields, including many applications in diabetology [93]. The evaluation of glycaemic control is particularly used in critical care units, where patients experience unpredictable and sudden metabolic changes, due to critical illness and/or clinical changes in nutritional support. These latter lead to highly-variable blood glucose levels, which can adversely affect clinical results and eventually lead to death [94]. Model-based control of glycaemia is widely employed in critical care, where the patient's environmental variables and inputs are better controlled. Metabolic system models include the pharmacokinetics of insulin and the pharmacodynamic interaction of glucose and insulin. The metabolic models can increase their accuracy and/or resolution by including specific patients' parameter.

Among the basic models used for clinical glycaemic control, the most famous one is the Minimal Model of Bergman et al. [95]. This simple model has two compartments for insulin pharmacokinetics and a third equation for insulin-glucose pharmacodynamics. By the way, every model that faces glycaemic metabolic control must consider these parameters: insulin pharmacokinetics and distribution, glucose pharmacokinetics and glucose-insulin pharmacodynamics descripting glucose elimination [94].

Most model-based glycaemic control requires a patient specific model, due to the variation between patients in insulin sensitivity and in other critical dynamic parameters. The main aim of glycaemic control is to maintain levels in an acceptable range. To this aim, a model, a glucose sensor and patient-specific parameter identification method are needed. The primary control input is the insulin administration, followed by modulating the nutritional input. Nevertheless, these models can be applied in clinical diagnosis in glucose tolerance and insulin sensitivity tests [96] and for self-management blood glucose therapy. Especially the simplest models, equally effective, require patient-specific physiological parameters combined with measured data, and already exist algorithms to predict and control glycaemic crisis. Even if, outside hospital environment, environment stimuli not considered into the model, play an important role. Some example are psychological factors, stress, depression, physical activity, which can significantly alter the glycaemic outcomes [97].

An emerging system for improving the BGC regulation is the Artificial Pancreas (AP), also referred to "closed loop glucose control". The AP includes a glucose sensor, control algorithms, and an insulin infusion device. The glucose sensor monitors the variability over time of BGC, in order to adjust the insulin dosage and to measure the efficacy of therapy after administration. However, the model needs an external input, such as meal announcement in advance, combined with feedback control to improve the glycaemia regulation [98].

Non-invasive methods for glucose monitoring and/or less invasive are more desirable alternatives than the above mentioned technology. One of the first attempt to apply bioimpedance measurement to non-invasive continuous glucose monitoring was carried out by the Cadduff's group in 2003 [99]. The sensor for impedance measurement had the size of a wristwatch and holed an open resonant circuit coupled to the skin and a circuit. Its clinical trials highlighted a good correlation between changes in blood glucose and sensors results. However, the main constraint was the calibration, with the patient unmoving for 60 min before the measurement. According to these studies, Pendragon Medical ltd of Switzerland, developed a commercial wrist-watch: Pendra, Fig. 1.11A [100]. The back of the watch had a tape that allowed the contact with the skin to perform impedance measurements through its open resonant circuit at (1 to 200) MHz. Unfortunately, once launched on the market, more than 30 % of the patients could not use the device, since their skin types and basic skin impedances were unsuitable. Overall, the measurements also showed poor correlation with conventional glucose meters and, therefore, the product was withdrawn from the market [101].

Another attempt, to use a "smart watch" as non-invasive glucose monitor, was the biographer GlucoWatch®, Fig. 1.11B, (Cygnus Inc.) [102]. The device extracts glucose concentrations through intact skin in interstitial fluid (ISF), where it is measured by an amperometric biosensor by reverse iontophoresis (RI). Clinical trials of the GlucoWatch showed adequate precision for home blood-glucose monitoring. However, the device was not designed to replace a regular blood glucose meter. Eventually, GlucoWatch was retracted from the market because of reported skin irritation caused by the RI process, the long necessary warm up time (2–3 h), and the need for calibration using standard blood glucose strips [103].

Considering the last failures, researchers need to focus on the production of reliable, efficient, and non-invasive glucose monitoring platforms. A proposal for a new device which exploits bioimpedance to assess insulin absorption is shown in next chapters.

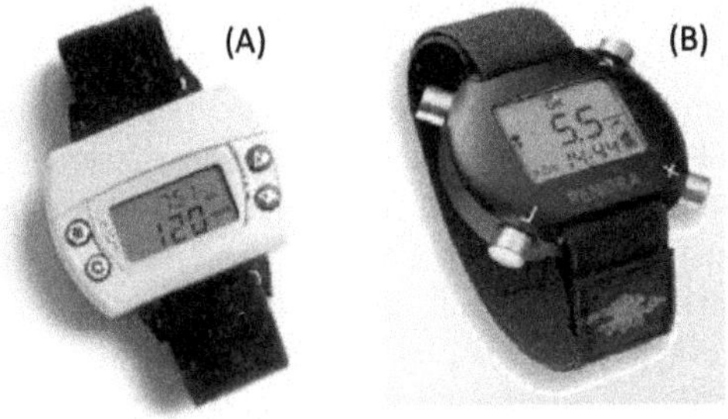

FIGURE 1.11
Pendra (A) and Glucowatch (B) -> Glucowatch (A) and Pendra (B).

1.3.2 Diet Planning Support

The study of body composition through bioimpedance techniques has aroused more and more interest not only for the clinical world, including nutrition and sports, but in all fields whose main goal is the achievement of a healthy lifestyle. The advantages of this method are highlighted by the speed of execution, safety and reduced impact on healthcare costs. In clinical practice, the primary purpose of body composition measurements is the evaluation of lean mass, and fat mass to assess nutritional status.

BIA is more sensitive than anthropometric measurements, which include body mass index (BMI), height, triceps skin fold, and abdominal circumference. Therefore, it is recommended for both hospitalized and outpatient nutritionally at risk patients [104]. In this case, BIA application is based on the capacity of hydrated tissues to conduct electrical energy. It is the most used method for evaluating body composition in the nutritional field.

In modern society, the increase in inactive population generates a constantly growth of overweight and obesity in both the adult and paediatric populations. Thus, the diet planning support, performed by a professional, is taking on a key role. In this scenario, the relationship between nutrition and clinic has become crucially important. Through bioimpedance and medical devices dedicated to measure the body composition, alterations in the state of health are brought out. Prevention interventions, capable of minimizing main risk factors, can be implemented, promoting suitable lifestyles for all ages. In this framework, BIA is a valuable ally in the assessment of body composition changes, in weight loss and, in special nutritional regimens, follow-up of training programs, evaluation and follow-up of body and weight-status development in paediatric age, and evaluation and control of the state of nutrition and hydration in pregnancy.

BIA allows tailored nutritional support in disease-specific therapy and it is crucial for diabetes patients. It ensures the optimization of nutritional intakes according to nutritional needs, since improper dietary intake can have profound metabolic effects. As already mentioned, BIA allows the evaluation of FM, and body fat is a core element of metabolic characteristics, including insulin resistance, and significant dangerous effects on diabetes and cardiovascular disease. Total adiposity and adipose tissue distribution are important determinants of insulin resistance and type-2 diabetes. A powerful relationship between insulin resistance and adiposity has been long recognized; indeed, adipose tissue distribution is an important factor of insulin resistance and type-2 diabetes, whose therapy includes diet planning [105, 106].

Each meal contains a different quantity of nutritious, such as water, carbohydrate, fat protein, glucose, vitamin, and minerals, which are absorbed in different ways by the gastro-intestinal system [107]. It is not easy to evaluate the glucose path through the intestine evaluating plasma glucose, since hepatic glucose balance, namely basal, varies significantly after food ingestion [108]. Thus, it is important to evaluate the effect of food on the glycaemic variability. The index to be taken into account is the Glycaemic Index (GI), a relative measure of the blood glucose raising potential of carbohydrate-rich foods and reflects carbohydrate quality [109]. Low-GI foods can improve blood glucose control in persons with diabetes. Glycaemic load (GL) is the product of carbohydrate content per serving of food and its GI. Low-GI and low-GL diets are associated with lower risk for type-2 diabetes and cardiovascular disease. On the other hand, also type-1 diabetes patients, who need for lifelong insulin treatments, should be taught to count carbohydrates, especially when they have to regulate the insulin dosage before each meal that is different from basal administration. Both for type-1 and type-2 diabetes patients it is important to collaborate with a team of experts in nutrition that can support them in planning the right diet.

BIA, especially in paediatric obesity could lead to a better understanding of the aetiology of obesity, and could help to establish preventive program for this disease. As matter of fact, between 1999 and 2004, the National Health and Nutrition Examination Survey program in United States included bioimpedance analysis to assess the health and nutritional status of adults and children due to its more reliability in evaluation FM and FFM, especially in subjects with higher amount of segmented fat.

Furthermore, another application of BIA is found in the units of cardiology, nephrology, oncology, and intensive care. In these units, monitoring the patient's nutritional and hydration status is a crucial evaluation to set up a correct therapeutic intervention, and an adequate nutritional strategy, aiming to reduce the clinical and functional consequences of the disease and the length of hospital stay. Thus, evaluation of BMI, FFM, and FM are increasingly used to evaluate nutritional status in hospitalized patients. During the hospital stay, the BIA is a great help for the evaluation of the water-electrolyte balance and protein metabolism in the patient undergoing artificial nutrition, in the acute and post-acute, intensive patient, and in general, in the critically ill patient with hydro-electrolytic and nutritional disorder. However, the injected currents do not interfere with the cardiac stimulation devices or pacemakers [104]. The body composition allows to assess the nutritional and clinical status of a patient, which is crucial in some diseases as cachexia to estimate the nature or overweightness and the degree of preservation of the muscle mass.

In clinical practice, it is important to control the ECW volume after total parenteral nutrition or to prevent its increase in case of malnutrition, sepsis or trauma. Weight lost and body cell mass depletion are important clinical parameters and complications for HIV patients or tumour cachexia or infection. Therefore, BIA is a suitable method for assessing body cell mass in these patients. Moreover, BIA may assist to document the response of nutrition support during patient's follow-up of numerous clinical conditions, such as surgery transplantation, Crohn's disease, cancer, and VIH/AIDS [110, 111].

Consequently, the diet planning to manage nutritionally at risk patient may reduce the clinical and practical outcomes of the diseases or the hospital recovery and healthcare cost [112].

Body composition is also an important factor to evaluate the volume distribution of many drugs, as well as in geriatrics and paediatrics and cancer patients. Indeed, the frequent assessment of body composition should be applied to personalize treatment doses according to the FFM and/or FM values of each subject. For example, loss of FFM could affect clinical outcome by decreasing the tolerance and efficacy of chemotherapy, being a significant predictor of chemotherapy toxicity. Since, the volume of distribution of chemotherapy drugs depends on the FFM, therefore, it is not possible to administer the same of the drugs in patients with FFM lower than normal, as it would increase the risk of toxicity [113–115].

BIA could guide physicians in the choice of nutritional therapies, the optimal drug dosage by improving so the efficacy-tolerance and cost-efficiency ratios of the therapeutical strategies.

Furthermore, BIA can be used in sports as significant diagnostic value; it can provide to professional athletes more precise and optimized tools to track changes in body composition reflecting the effectiveness of the training and guide the athlete's evolution towards better performance, while preserving the state of health.

In fact, in the landscape of the 21st century, we are witnessing both a demographic and epidemiological transformation. The progressive aging of the population and a reduced prevalence of infectious diseases in favour of an expansion of chronic degenerative diseases, a more sedentary lifestyle, also linked to the increase of remote working, are generating an increase in the socio-economic burden linked to care costs, assistance and social security. Following this change, it is necessary to provide non-invasive solutions, more effective and with a reduced impact on healthcare costs, designed ad hoc for the management of the critical patient and for the control of the state of vulnerability, and BIA is one of these solutions.

1.4 Bioimpedance Measurements in Orthopaedics

Orthopaedics is a branch of medicine that studies the musculoskeletal system and the pathologies associated with this system. The musculoskeletal system is represented by the musculoskeletal apparatus, by the tendons and ligaments and by the peripheral nerves that move in these organs.

Our body is made up of 68 joints which represent the connections between the various bones. Ligaments and capsules are essential in the joints because they ensure their stability. Joints can be simple (making rough movements) or large (making fine/precise movements). The tendons connect the bones to the muscles which contracting/stretching generates movement between the bones.

Peripheral nerves can have sensory, motor, or mixed function (both of the above). The tasks of the nerves is to detect the information signaled (perception) by the parts of the musculoskeletal system and to send it to the medulla. The latter sends information to the cerebral cortex and waits for the response (movement) to be sent to the nerves.

The main task of orthopaedics is to treat joint pathologies, but to a lesser extent it also deals with fractures and prosthetic implants.

Common orthopaedic pathologies include osteitis, tumours, dislocations, ruptured ligaments or ruptured tendons, bruises and osteoarthritis.

Traumatology is a branch of orthopaedics that studies the damage to parts of the human body (external or internal) due to exogenous violent actions (mechanical action, thermal action, or chemical action). As will be dealt with specifically in the next subsection, the trauma can be defined direct trauma if it causes the injury at the point of application of the exogenous force. While the trauma can be considered indirect trauma if it causes the injury at some distance from the point of application of the exogenous force. The main objective is to detect the best way to intervene on the lesion and restore the integrity of the injured part, or to replace the injured part with a prosthesis. The injuries reported by subjects range from mild injuries (cuts, abrasions) to more serious ones (bone fractures, damage to organs and tissues). The nature of the trauma, the extent of the exogenous force, the complications caused by the injury and the body part affected must be considered to obtain an accurate diagnosis of the injury.

A separate consideration must be made for sport orthopaedics and traumatology, which requires greater diagnostic accuracy and greater timeliness of treatment to allow the athlete to return to previous competitive skills and to avoid possible relapses or worsening.

The established techniques in these fields for patient diagnosis and care are expensive and risky. For example, radiography is the most used diagnostic technique, because it requires little time and no preliminary preparation of the patient. However, the patient is subjected to considerable radiation exposure, which with a low probability, could cause cancer.

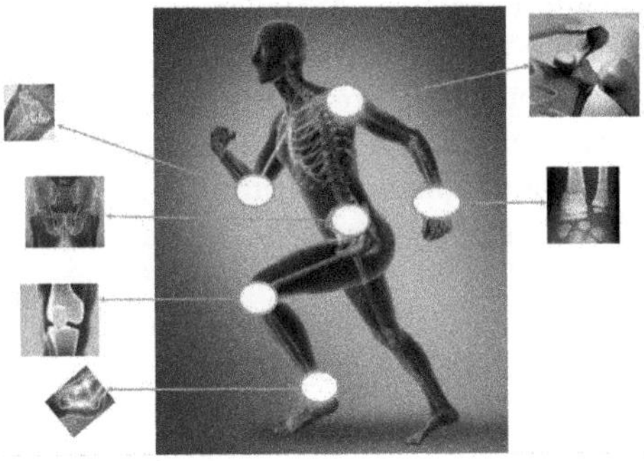

FIGURE 1.12
Some possible trauma in the human body.

The analysis of electrical bioimpedance is a technique that could replace the techniques already validated, because it is non-invasive and non-destructive [116].

The applicability of this analysis in the trauma field is manifold. In fact, it can be used for the predictive diagnosis of the outcome of a trauma, to evaluate the state of health of the bones and cartillage, to monitor the effect of the injection of a drug on the electrical properties of the tissues under exam and to monitor the growth state of the tissues surrounding a prosthesis [117].

With regard to the tissues surrounding a prosthesis, the problem is that it starts to proliferate and must withstand the mechanical stresses of the device. Consequently, the quality of this contact is decisive for the usefulness of the system. There are several clinical methods to study contact stability, such as radiology or acoustic resonance. However, there are critical problems in both methods that could be solved with BIA. Radiology is an invasive technique that does not allow the evaluation of soft tissues in the first analysis. While acoustic resonance is not an effective method for deep prostheses.

Moreover, Yoshida et al., confirmed the validity of the electrical impedance measurement for the evaluation of fracture fixation [118]. This analysis allowed to clarify the behaviour at the interface of fixation bone [118]. It allows to monitor the growth of the surrounding tissues (which is very difficult with radiology) and the variation of their electrical properties.

About the predictive diagnosis of a trauma, a smart and wearable devise was realized, by Lin et al., to detect pressure of lesions of the tissues surrounding the internal cavities and to monitor the changes in the tissues [119]. In the following study, the bioimpedance spectroscopy was used to create visual maps to monitor damaged tissue areas at risk of complications.

Finally, the bioimpedance spectroscopy can be a decisive solution for monitoring the health of joints such as the knee joint. The need for this analysis is due to the quality of our joints, which determine the quality of our life and excessive pain could cause significant complications [11]. Moreover, BIA appears to be an optimal choice in the creation of personalized therapies for this joint. As already mentioned previously, the BIA allows to monitor the spread of drugs under the skin [117]; in addition, it can provide information to identify the duration of action of the drug [120]. The problem with this type of analysis is the uncertainty arising from the differences in physical characteristics of individuals and from the variability of these characteristics in the same individual over time [11]. This problem that can be treated with a Finite Element Method (FEM) model of the joint that integrates the muscokeletal parameters of the subjects. In this way, it is possible to compensate for the different sources of uncertainty (such as emotional state, temperature) and obtain a more accurate impedance [11].

1.4.1 Trauma Outcome Assessment

The possibility to evaluate skeletal muscle health status, mass or volume, in an effective and accurate way is advantageous in different medical application. It might also facilitate the diagnosis process, assessing surgical outcomes, monitoring growth and development both in healthy and with chronic disease patients. The most accurate diagnostic methods used in clinical practice to evaluate muscle mass are expensive, time consuming and not totally risk-free. Moreover they are not handy for routine use due to the inaccessibility and prohibitive cost. On the other side, cheaper methods such as anthropometry, dealing with measurements of the size, weight and proportion of the human body and skeleton, present limited accuracy. Therefore, an alternative approach is the bioelectrical impedance analysis. In this specific case, by measuring impedance and specific resistivity of tissues it can estimate limb muscle volume, and is relevant in evaluation of impairments of muscle function in neurological disease or trauma [121].

Trauma to soft tissues badly affects fluid distribution and cell structure. Skeletal muscle injuries can be classified as indirect and direct. Indirect injuries, including muscles strain or soreness, result from an abrupt passive muscle elongation or overload. On the other hand, direct injuries are usually a result of external trauma and can provoke simple contusion or even muscle failure, according to trauma force and the muscles state of contraction. Another classification takes into account the severity of injury, by evaluating the involved amount of muscle fibres. They range from grade I to grade III. In grade I, the discomfort or the loss of movement is minimal, since the only few muscles fibers are damaged. In grade III, the muscles function is almost loss and the tear extending across the entire cross-section of the muscle.

The primary imaging technique used by clinicians to evaluate the type, the severity and the muscles involved in the injury is the Magnetic Resonance Imaging (MRI), even if it is expensive and time consuming [122]. On the other side, localized BIA measurements of muscle groups allows the detection of soft tissue injury and its severity. Localized BIA affords a safe, non-invasive and practical method for determine skeletal muscle mass or volume and assessing perturbations in it, since the pathological and physiological changes are connected to tissues electrical variables. Therefore, localized BIA can be used before, after injury and, during recovery, for monitoring clinical treatments progress. It recognizes different degrees of muscle injury according to changes in BIA variables. Muscles injuries commonly affect athletes and represent between 10 % and 55 % of all sports injuries. In particular, skeletal muscle injuries constitute the majority of sports-related injuries, as an illustration muscle injuries constituted 31 % of all injuries in football players, and 92 % of all injuries affect the 4 big muscle groups in the lower limbs. Hence, prevention of muscle injuries, reduction of recovery time and re-injury rate, monitoring of recovery, evaluation of best time for return to game, are important challenges in sport medicine [123]. Also another study evidences the potential utility of localized BIA as a practical tool in the follow-up of muscle injury in soccer players, describing the changes in BIA values in response to different muscle injury and different grade [124].

Another application in sport medicine is represented by multi-frequency BIA. It enables instantly assessment of skeletal muscle in terms of anatomical, physiological, and pathological state, by making possible to analyze the entire muscle or reach muscle fibre. The use of multi-frequency BIA parameters and their combination can be exploited to detect contralateral muscle loss, extracellular fluid differences, contracted state, and cell transport/metabolic activity, which relate to muscle performance. Thus, this technique is easily applicable in the clinic or sports setting [125].

Considering another kind of trauma, the pressure ulcers, impedance spectroscopy is used to detect and monitor surface and fracture wounds. Ulcers can affect the quality of life of many individuals, they are areas of soft tissue breakdown that result from sustained mechanical loading of the skin and underlying tissues, so not only skin tissue, but also muscle tissue may be very vulnerable to mechanical loading. This pressure interferes with blood flow, thus causing the skin to break down and form an ulcer. Moreover, skin ulceras are common in diabetic patients, and BIA can monitor and describe cellular changes during the heal of skin ulceras.

In [126], a non-invasive electrical device is developed in order to detect pressure-induced tissue damage in a human patients using impedance spectroscopy. The benefits of using impedance spectroscopy are proven to detect pressure ulcers, and early detection of tissue damage. Injured skeletal muscle, along with ligaments and tendons, undergoes process of break, inflammation, degeneration and fibrosis. An early response to muscular trauma is inflammation and hematoma which fills the gap of the disrupted muscles post-trauma. Structural damage of the muscle fibers usually heals with formation of scar tissue. The most common muscle injuries include delayed-onset muscle soreness, muscular contusion, muscular strain, and muscular laceration. Among these types of injuries, the mechanism of injury, pathologic changes, treatment, and outcome vary greatly.

BIA systems represent portable and effective devices for quantifying knee joint health, following an acute injury both inside hospital and outside the clinic and a valuable help in rehabilitation process and monitoring. The ability of BIA to assess knee injury relys on the sensitivity of the system to detect even the smallest changes in interstitial fluid volume. As example, in [127], the authors exploit a wearable BIA device, composed by a band with 4 electrodes placed around the knee joint. They inject a sinusoidal current of 2 mA at a frequency of 50 kHz, and declared that the knee resistance of all the injured subjects was lower than healthy ones. The system was able to measure knee impedance and provide information about knee joint edema and injury, together with longitudinal changes during recovery. In fact, the same device was used to detect knee edema enabling high-resolution, and quantitative assessment of both the structural and hemodynamic characteristics of the knee joint [128].

Edema is an abnormal accumulation of extracellular water resulting from malfunction of the physiologic mechanisms. It represents also the lymphatic system reaction to intracellular pathogens or tissues and cell damaged by a trauma. Post-traumatic edema of lower limbs is characterized by long-lasting swelling of the limb, erythema, and increased skin temperature at the site of injury. Knee edema is a normal body response to the surgical trauma caused by total knee arthroplasty. Bioelectrical impedance measurements may be a convenient, safe, quick, non-invasive and not hampered by scars and medications to measure muscular mass and edema after knee arthroplasty. Edema generates an increase in limb fluid volume that cause a change in impedance values. In particular, BIA allows the estimation of limb extracellular and intracellular fluid and the total fluid [129].

The monitoring of fluid volume is crucial also for people with trans-tibial limb loss using prostheses. Since people with limb loss usually experience residual limb volume changes that influence the optimum fit of their prosthesis, the identification of patients characteristic and their residual limb fluid volume may help for identifying and ranking prosthetic design features.

1.4.2 Bone Health Status Assessment

Bone fractures can occur under traumatic event or non-traumatic condition such as osteoporosis, arthritis, bone cancer and so on.

Nowadays, the oldest but the most common technique used to diagnose fractured bones, joint dislocations, injuries and joint abnormalities is X-ray Radiography. This exam requires little time and no special preparation, but bulky and expensive equipment. In spite of the use of a very-small dose of ionizing radiation to produce pictures of any bone in the body, there is an accumulative effect of the ionizing radiation that lead to a slight chance of cancer from excessive exposure to radiation. Moreover, pregnant women should avoid this procedure. In order to overcome the limitation of X-Ray radiography, BIA could represent an innovative approach to detect bone health status [130].

However, BIA measurements can exploit different electrodes configurations. The first author to study tissues properties was Gabriel, in her in-vitro and ex-vivo studies she used BIA with different electrodes configuration to characterize conductivity and permittivity of biological tissues of several species, including human bones [131]. In particular, bone tissue is a mineralized and viscous-elastic connective tissue, which plays important functions in our body such as support and protection of organs. Bone tissue consists mainly of two types within the same specific bone: trabecular (cancellous) and cortical (compact). Both, according to their different microstructure, present differences in their dependency on frequency. In particular, dielectric parameters of cancellous bone, especially relative permittivity and dissipation factor, are specifically connected to a trabecular microstructure as shown in [132]. Thus, electrical and dielectric parameters of trabecular bone, might deliver important diagnostic parameters not considered in bone mineral density measurements. Moreover, not only the microscopic composition, but also measurement variables such as frequency and orientation affect the electrical properties of cancellous and cortical bone differently [133]. This electric and dielectric parameters could be used not only for detection of bone quality in-vitro but also in special cases of open orthopaedic surgery. For example, during total joint replacement procedure, BIA might provide a tool for fast quantitative diagnostics of bone grafts quality or bone health status.

Another medical application of BIA is maxilo-facial surgery such as proposed by [116]. Ex-vivo studies on bovine bone, emulating the insert of dental implant into bone, were conducted to evaluate the proper osteo-integration of implants by means of a suitable model and an effective measurement technique. BIA measurements were carried out on two metallic dental implants, placed into the bone, in low-frequency range of 10 Hz to 65 kHz, with amplitude range of the sine-wave stimulus of 10–100 mV using with an impedance analyzer (Solartron 1250).

A similar approach has been used to study fracture healing and new bone formation. To treat human open fractures of tibia might be used external fixators, these latter used as invasive electrodes to evaluate the healing biological process [134]. The femur or thigh bone is the largest bone of the human body and its fracture proximal can lead to dislocation of the fracture ends and related hip problems. Surgical treatment of hip fracture includes surgical implants to fix the ends of the femur in their anatomical correct position to enable healing. The hip joint is classified as a ball socket joint; it is formed by the articulation of the femoral head and the acetabulum through a synovial join. Thus, hip implants used in total hip replacements are made up of a socket-like shell that is surgically inserted into the acetabulum of the pelvis, and a ball-like device to replace the femoral head and a prosthesis fixed in the femoral bone with the bone cement. The composition of the surgical implants is widely different, generally made of titanium, cobalt and chromium, or newest composite, or other materials such as ceramics and hydroxyapatites. These materials can eventually increase or decrease the electrical conductance and thus affect impedance measurements. Thus, BIA measurement at single frequency 50 kHz has been used to characterize hip fracture and hip replacement surgery [135].

Meanwhile, BIA has been used to evaluate osseonitegration of hip prosthesis implants. In particular, this in an innovative electrical approach to characterize the quality of the bone-prosthesis interface. Monitoring this complex biological process, especially during the first recovery weeks' post-implant, is important to evaluate the success of the surgery. Since the clinical success over the time of the surgical procedure relies on the stability of the implants, the metallic or composite prostheses must be firmly anchored to residual bone by specific cement and by the interface tissue resulted of osseointegration [136]. The same approach can be also used to evaluate cochlear implants, which are surgically implanted neuroprosthetic device, usually in titanium, that is inserted into the skull fixed through osseointegression, to treat deafness and severe hearing loss [137].

Another application of BIA analyzes and compares bioimpedance parameters observed in the knees of healthy and with osteoarthritis, helping so physicians in disease diagnosis. Osteoarthritis is one of the most important muskoskeletal disorder and one of the leading cause of disability worldwide involving one out of every four adults and with a financial burden of billions of dollars in health costs. Osteoarthritis is a degenerative process involving all of the major joint tissues, including articular cartilage, synovium, and subchondral bone. Osteoarthritis is the most common form of arthritis. It is strongly associated with aging and typically affects the knee and hip and radiographic imaging is normally used for its diagnostic and monitoring. However, bioimpedance parameters have been proven to be sensitive to the physiological changes associated with osteoarthritis. Then, the BIA technique, the electrical modelling and the parameter evaluation might provide an objective and non-invasive tool for assisting in the diagnosis of knee osteoarthritis and a promising tool for objective and long-term patient follow up [138].

In conclusion, bioimpedance measurements have the potentialities to satisfy clinical need for an easy, non-ionizing, low cost, quick and portable instruments to detect bone fractures, wherever pre-hospital care is called to operate and to monitor bone healing and advance in personalized healthcare.

Part II

Methods and Instrumentation

2

Measurement Method for Aesthetic Medicine

CONTENTS

Transdermal drug delivery is widely appreciated in aesthetic medicine. As a matter of fact, it guarantees less systemic uptake and no skin irritation with respect to oral administration and hypodermic injection. However, the amount of drug penetrating the skin during aesthetic treatments strongly depends on individual characteristics. At present, there are no standardized methods for measuring the drug delivered in-vivo and non invasively. This chapter focuses on a method for assessing non-invasively the drug under the skin, based on impedance spectroscopy.

DOI: 10.1201/9781003170143-2

2.1 Measurements Concepts for Aesthetic Medicine

The development of transdermal drug delivery is providing new techniques to target site-specific delivery and to enhance skin penetration. Hence, it allows to extend the range of therapeutic and aesthetic compounds that can be delivered through the skin. Transdermal drug delivery guarantees less systemic uptake and no skin irritation with respect to oral administration and hypodermic injection. For this reason, it is greatly appreciated in aesthetic medicine. Several strategies are well-estabilished in transdermal delivery: i.e., chemical-enhancers, electroporation, and iontophoresis [139, 140]. All these methods are proved to enhance the penetration of the drug under the skin in ex-vivo laboratory studies. Currently, however, the amount of drug actually passed through the skin cannot be assessed in vivo and non-invasively [141, 142].

Individual features (e.g., age, sex, emotions, and so on) deeply impact on skin permeability and, consequently, on the amount of delivered drug. An accurate measurement of the penetrated drug could allow more effective personalized treatments, in the contest of the advanced concepts of personalized medicine [143].

Thus far, available measurement methods have several problems that make their clinical application very complex. Indeed, these methods are invasive and time-consuming; moreover, they require expensive equipment, and not allow the deep skin layers analysis.

An effective solution to these problems is bioimpedance spectroscopy (BIS), owing to its minimal invasiveness. BIS is already widely used in biomedical research and clinical practice, especially in dermatology, as discussed in Chapter 1.

Strictly speaking, a tissue is a collection of similar cells specialised to fulfil a specific function. The cells lie in a supporting framework, called matrix, made of materials produced also by surrounding cells. The physiological behaviour of a cell is defined both by internal elements and parameters, as well as by external factors, namely the extracellular fluid. The fluid is often secreted by cells to provide a constant environment for cellular operations; thus, it has the same composition of intracellular fluid, but with a different concentration. This fluid is circulated throughout the body along with the blood, in the spaces between blood vessel and tissues, where material exchange occurs by diffusion. The body fluid is mainly a water solution with ions and other substances [144]. Therefore, a human tissue can be approximated to an electrolyte solution containing a large amount of cells. In conductometry, the quantity of a conductive substance (solute) dissolved in a solution can be estimated from the variation of solution resistance. In fact, the equivalent conductance of the solution also depends on how much solute is actually present.

The electrolyte is a ionic conducting medium, whereas, in the case of solutions, the solute is dissolved in the solvent and participates to the conductive properties of the solution as whole. Information on the state of particles in a solution, their actual size, mobility, and association, can be obtained applying quite rigorous theories and model representations. In particular, the electrical conductance of electrolyte solutions can be measured with a high degree of precision at low concentrations. Analogously, a biological tissue can be studied by impedance measurements because it is characterized by ionic conductivity and dielectric relaxation phenomena.

BIA allows to obtain useful information about changes occurred under the skin; in particular by referring to the variation of impedance measured during the pre- and post-drug administration phases. Therefore, the first purpose of this chapter is to illustrate a method for assessing the quantity of a conductive substance delivered into a tissue, by analyzing the variation of tissue impedance caused by the substance. The main challenge is the identification of the relationship between the impedance variation and the administrated quantity. The second purpose is to illustrate the method application in the field of the aesthetic medicine. To this aim, a preliminary experimental campaign is presented for proving the feasibility of the assessment method and identifying the bandwidth of interest. Then, further experiments are presented for:

1. validating the proposed method;
2. performing a metrological characterization;
3. and optimizing the metrological performance.

The tests are carried out initially on a human tissue emulator. Among many vegetables and fruits already electrically characterized, the eggplant is chosen for the reasons reported below. Firstly, the eggplant exhibits an electrical behaviour very similar to the human skin. Indeed, eggplants pulp can be modelled as an electrical circuit with concentrated parameters similar to those widely used for human tissue [145, 146]. Moreover, it was preferred to other vegetables, i.e., potato or carrot, for its porous structure and for its easy penetrability with a needle. Indeed, when the drug is injected in the potato, for example, it comes out immediately even using a 100 μl insulin needle. Finally, fruits were excluded due to the high presence of liquids and, therefore, the too low impedance with respect to human tissue.

2.2 Method

The method, illustrated here for measuring the amount of drug actually conveyed under the skin, is based on the following main phases (Fig. 2.1):

- A known amount of drug is administered into the tissue under test; this generates a corresponding measurable change in the impedance magnitude of the tissue. Once generated a sinusoidal current at a given frequency, the impedance spectroscopy allows to acquire the corresponding voltage drop through the electrodes and the signal conditioning stage.

- Impedance spectroscopy initially calculates both the spectral response for all the frequency into the bandwidth, and the relative change in impedance at a fixed frequency. The impedance spectrum is then employed during a classification phase to recognize the peculiarities of the tissue under investigation. The relative change in impedance is employed during an inverse modelling phase to calculate the amount of drug through suitable coefficients, identified by the tissue classification.
- A preliminary impedance measurement allows to obtain information on the properties of the tissue under test and its characteristics; these latter influence the sensitivity of the measurement. The reproducibility is enhanced by this preliminary impedance measurement, which improves intra- and inter-individual measurement reproducibility;
- The electrodes, placed on the tissue under test, are essential for carrying out the measurement. However, the progressive penetration of their electrolytic gel into the tissue causes a corresponding decrease in the impedance over time. Therefore, the impedance stability needs to be monitored in a proper time interval;
- Finally, the measured amount of drug, penetrating into the tissue under test, is estimated by a linear relationship to the impedance variation.

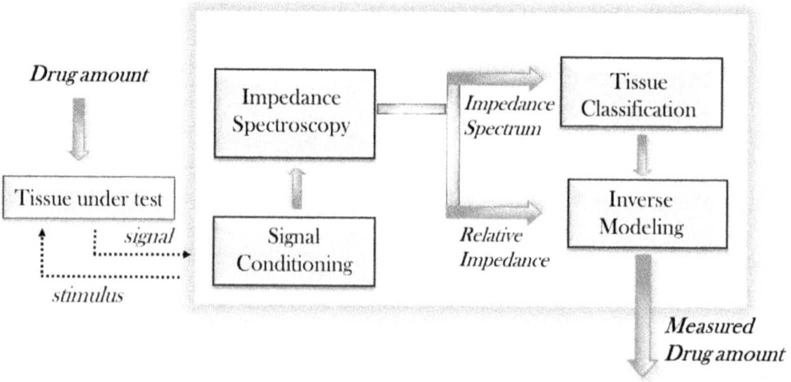

FIGURE 2.1
Measurement method phases.

A linear model, despite its simplicity, is candidate to adequately express the relationship between the amount of injected substance and the variation in the impedance magnitude. In order to mitigate the impact of the initial conditions and the common-mode noise, the percentage variation with respect to the initial value is set as the output of the measurement method.

Moreover, in a first approximation, this allows to not consider the specific skin bio-dynamics and, thus, results in improving the measurement reproducibility at varying the individual and inter-individual skin characteristics.

The amount of drug actually penetrated into the tissue is measured by assessing the difference between the impedance spectrum before and after administration. The measurement instrument is based on standard off-the-shelf components. The spectroscope ensures an accuracy of 5 % in its operating bandwidth of 50 kHz, and it complies with the safety rules for biomedical devices [147].

2.3 Feasibility

Experimentation is the best known way to test the veracity of scientific theories; in the following sections, the feasibility of the illustrated measurement method is evaluated. Therefore, the experimental setup and the results of the exploratory campaign are presented and discussed.

2.3.1 Setup

Seven eggplants were peeled and cut in rectangular-shaped pulp blocks 40 mm × 40 mm × 100 mm of the same size. Impedance spectroscopy is performed at room temperature using a Solartron 1260A Impedance Analyzer (Solartron Analytical, Hampshire, UK) [148] with a frequency range from 10 μHz to 32 MHz. The Solartron uses powerful microprocessor-controlled digital and analog techniques to provide fast and accurate measurements over a wide frequency range.

Impedance analyzers usually utilize the voltamperometric method to measure the unknown impedance. By applying the Ohm law, the impedance is calculated by injecting a known current and by measuring the resulting voltage drop. Among the different ways to connect the object under test, the two-terminal configuration is selected by considering both the negligible effect of parasitic capacitance and the expecting medium impedance levels in the interest bandwidth. The methods to connect the tissue under test to the impedance analyzer vary both with the material and the shape of the target tissue. The contact resistance, arising between the contacts of the analyzer and the tissue under test, is unstable and varies with factors including surface roughness, electrode wear, and contact pressure. With the purpose of mitigating the impact of contact resistance on the measurements, pre-gelled electrodes with one of the largest surfaces on the market (7.28 cm^2) are selected. The electrodes

PG 500 FIAB [149], specific for bioimpedance analysis, are used with medical adhesive solid gel biocompatible and a low impedance conductive paper aluminium, in order to get good electrical contact. The highly-flexible material of the electrodes allows their easy positioning, and the gel sticks easily to the numerous diverse skins and peculiar curves of the human body. Despite the strong adherence, electrodes are effortlessly taken off and are non-irritating to delicate skin. An electrodes gap of 4.6 cm is selected, in order to ensure the right penetration of the current lines for the tissue under test.

A commercial drug, which can be electrically compared to drug used in aesthetic medicine such as the hyaluronic acid, is used. It has a conductivity of 526 μS/cm and its content is: water, sodium acrylates copolymer, hyrogated polydecene, PPG-1Trideceth-6, phosphatidylcoline, urea sorbitol, glycerin, and butylene glycol. The drug is injected 2 cm below the surface for the following volumes: 0.4 ml, 0.8 ml, and 1.2 ml. Meanwhile, a sinusoidal current of 1 mA is applied to the electrodes, and the corresponding voltage drop is measured in the frequency range of 1 Hz to 10 MHz, by a logarithmic frequency sweep of 10 steps/decade. After the preparation of the eggplant and the electrode application, the impedance spectrum is measured before the injection and after each of the three aforementioned doses.

2.3.2 Results

The tests were carried out according to the previously described experimental conditions. A linear relationship between the amount of injected drug and the impedance magnitude for each explored frequency is found. This result is expressed by means of Bode diagrams: graphical representations of the frequency responses, of magnitude and phase, using the logarithmic frequency scale. In Fig. 2.2, the plot (a) highlights that the increase of the amount of injected drug produces a related progressive decrease in impedance magnitude. In Fig. 2.2 (b), the phase trend does not show the same regularity.

The experiments were conducted in different conditions, by varying the eggplants, electrodes area and gap, the signal amplitude and frequency, as well as the conducting drugs.

Generally, in biomedical application of impedance spectroscopy, especially in dermatology, measurement uncertainty is mainly linked to electrode/electrolyte interface [150] and, therefore, to the skin hydration, electrode adhesion, humidity, temperature, and so on. During impedance measurement of intact human skin, at low frequency, the presence of the stratum corneum makes negligible the effect of electrode/electrolyte interface.

Unfortunately, in the peeled eggplants, the lack of a layer analogous to the corneum makes the above-mentioned uncertainty sources not negligible. Consequently, in Fig. 2.2, we can see a fluctuation of impedance and phase in the range of 150 Hz to 1000 Hz arising from the above-mentioned uncertainty sources.

Nonetheless, the effect related to the electrode/electrolyte interface is deterministic, because phenomena of alteration of the measured value (drift) can be modelled and, therefore, handled. These phenomena do not affect significantly the highlighted relationship between amount of drug and impedance magnitude. So, according to these results, in order to evaluate the amount of drug a simple impedance measurement can be used at a single frequency rather than a spectrum analysis over the whole bandwidth, which may not add further information.

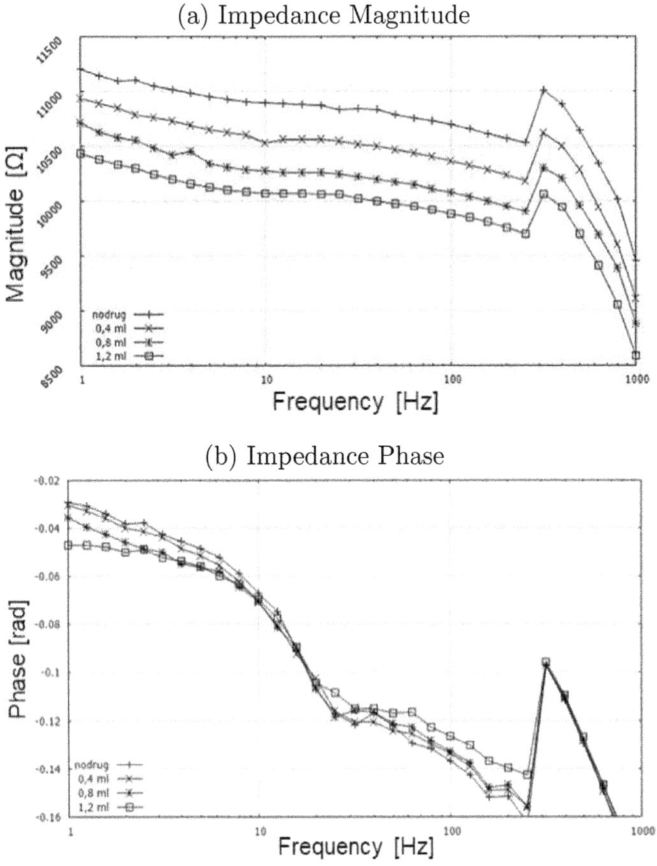

FIGURE 2.2
Impedance of eggplant pulp at varying the injected amount: Bode diagrams of impedance magnitude (a) and impedance phase (b) [2].

2.4 Validation

A further analysis of validation is needed to prove that the illustrated method is acceptable and ready to obtain reliable results. In the following, the setup and the results for the validation are illustrated.

2.4.1 Setup

For the validation experiment, again rectangular-shaped pulp samples of 40 mm × 40 mm × 100 mm eggplants peeled and cut are used. All the experiments follow the same procedure: in particular, it is assured the same preparation time for each eggplant and the same electrode application. Subsequently, the drug is injected 2 cm below the surface in volume concentration steps of: 0.2 ml, 0.4 ml, 0.6 ml, 0.8 ml, and 1.0 ml. In this case, all the measures are carried out by a calibrated Agilent 4263B LCR Meter [151] according to the conditions shown in Tab. 2.1. In particular, a signal amplitude of 20 mV is used for improving the linearity; meanwhile, the frequency of 1 kHz is selected, in order to mitigate electrode influence more relevant at low frequency. For filtering the random noise, 60 measurements are averaged. Finally, the electrodes gap is selected by evaluating the ideal condition of current depth within the tissue. The other parameters presented in the table will be extensively discussed in the following sections.

2.4.2 Results

The typical linear relation between percentage variation of impedance magnitude and drug amount, pointed out in Fig. 2.3, is confirmed also in these results. The linear relation between the amount of drug and the percentage impedance variation is achieved by normalizing the pre-injection drug value. In particular, it was experienced that by increasing the amount of drug with higher conductivity, the measured equivalent impedance decreased accordingly.

2.5 Metrological Characterization

In this book, the terminology of the international vocabulary of metrology (VIM) [152] is adopted. The method is characterized metrologically by employing the in-vitro experimental setup described previously. In particular, different parameters are analyzed, namely, the drift, the sensitivity, the nonlinearity, the repeatability, the accuracy, and the resolution.

TABLE 2.1
Metrological condition and results in the metrological characterization.

Parameter	**Drug conductivity**	**Signal Frequency**	**Electrodes Area**	**Electrode Gap**	**Signal Amplitude**
Value	666 μS/cm	1.00 kHz	3.64 cm^2	4.6 cm	20 mV
Characteristic	**Sensitivity** [ml^{-1}]	**Nonlinearity** [%]	**1-σ Repeatability** [%]	**Accuracy** [%]	**Resolution** [ml]
Value	3.8	0.47	0.07	0.68	0.05

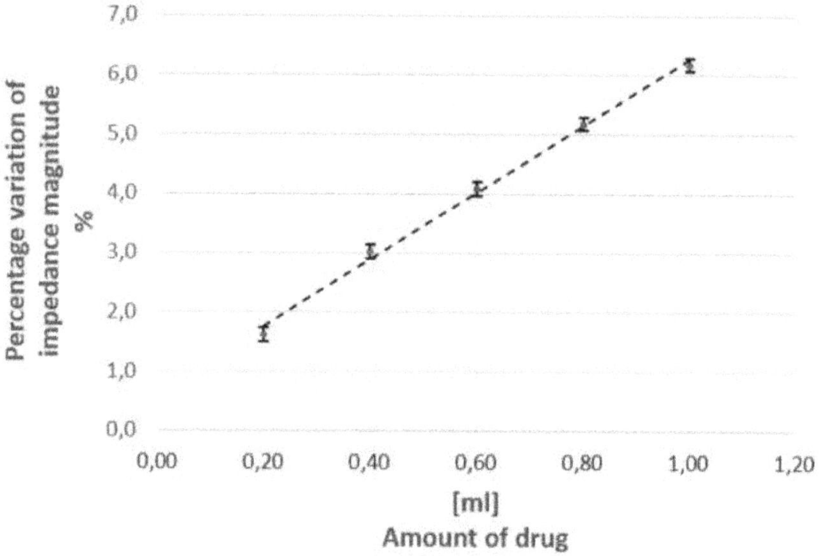

FIGURE 2.3
Impedance magnitude percentage variation vs drug amount in laboratory experiments [2].

2.5.1 Drift Analysis

The measurement of the amount of drug penetrating the skin during aesthetic treatments can be affected by different uncertainty sources; among them, the drift plays a significant role. Drift refers to continuous or incremental change in measurements over time due to changes in the metrological properties of a measuring instrument, or reference material [152].

It is further well known that the impedance of the skin is governed by the stratum corneum, especially at lower frequency; an increase in the hydration state will alter the electrical properties of the skin over time, and so the impedance significantly. The altered impedance response can most likely be attributed to the introduction of more charge carriers into the stratum corneum, due to a solution or gel penetration. The penetration of these ions can decrease the impedance of the skin layers [153].

Other aspects to consider are firstly, the gel might include other substances which can increase the penetration of the solvents into the stratum corneum and, subsequently, lower the impedance further. Secondly, the gel and electrodes occlude the passive water transport; moreover, the fluid accumulation produced under the electrodes can influence the measurements even further [153].

In in-vitro experiments based on eggplants, valid substitute for human skin without stratum corneum, the drift arises due to twofold main causes [154]. On one hand, the water evaporation contained into the eggplants prevents the creation of conductive channels for ions, and thus increases the impedance. On the other hand, the electrodes degradation, and the subsequent electrolyte gel penetration with high concentration of ions within the eggplants, significantly alters conduction process and lower the impedance. Therefore, the drift impact on the impedance measurement is to be assessed by a specific experimental analysis described below.

Five different eggplants samples were observed, and the impedance measurements recorded for a total time frame of 10^4 s. The results, presented in Fig. 2.4, show an initially decrease in the equivalent impedance magnitude: the drift is more affected by the electrolyte gel penetration than by the water evaporation. As a matter of fact, the electrolyte gel penetration increases the sample conductivity. Thus, the equivalent impedance magnitude lowers. After half an hour, the effect of water evaporation is more relevant and the impedance begins to increase. The drift effect is limited to far below 1 %, namely 0.4 %, upon 15 minutes after the electrodes application.

The drift impact on the experimental measurements can be assessed also by considering the measurement protocol and its specific times. A typical protocol in aesthetic medicine includes the administration of 5 consecutive drug doses, after the electrodes application, for a total time of 3 min. After each drug administration, 10 impedance measurements are carried out; each measurement require 1 s, so all the measurements are carried out in 10 s. Then, the 10 results are processed and the average and the standard deviation are calculated. The operator administers the new dose in 10 s. Thus, such a protocol makes reasonable to assume that the drift does not affect the measurement accuracy.

2.5.2 Sensitivity

The sensitivity represents the quotient of the variation of a measuring system response and the corresponding variation of a value of a measured quantity [152]. In this case, the instrument sensitivity is assessed as the slope of the linear regression model of the impedance magnitude variation and the amount of drug injected within eggplants. Its value in the above experiment is 3.8 ml^{-1} (Fig. 2.5).

For a typical dose of 10 ml of injected drug, a corresponding percentage variation of 38 % in impedance magnitude is observed, compared to the reference value of tissue impedance measured before the injection.

2.5.3 Nonlinearity

The sensitivity is assessed on the assumption of a linear model; thus, the error linked to this assumption is determined by one-way ANalysis Of VAriance

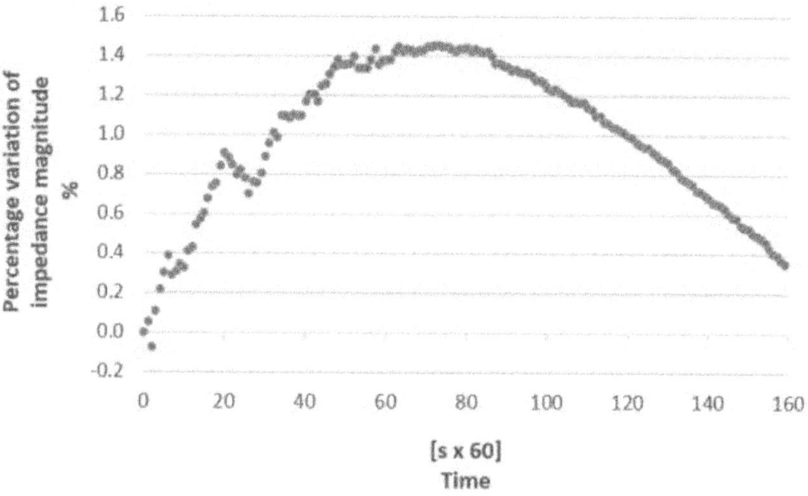

FIGURE 2.4
Measurement drift due to eggplant evaporation and electrode gel permeation [2].

(ANOVA) [155]. In particular, it is calculated as the residual standard deviation of the linear regression model, namely the nonlinearity. The typical value achieved in the above experiment is 0.47 %.

2.5.4 Repeatability

Repeatability describes the closeness of the agreement between repeated measurements of the same quantity, carried out in the same place, by the same person, on the same equipment, in the same way, at similar times [152].

In Fig. 2.6, the 1-σ repeatability of the above experiment is plotted; it is assessed as the percentage variation relative to the initial impedance value, at varying the amount of injected drug. A typical value of 0.07 % is determined.

2.5.5 Accuracy

Accuracy is the closeness of the agreement between measurement result and the conventional true value of a measurand [152]. In Fig. 2.7, it is assessed as the percentage deterministic error, and plotted in function of the injected drug.

A typical accuracy value of less than a few percent is achieved by averaging the maximum values in the above experiment. A calibration establishes the reliability of the instrument and ensures that its measurements are consistent. In this way, the error might be compensated by computing its value for a specific measurement configuration.

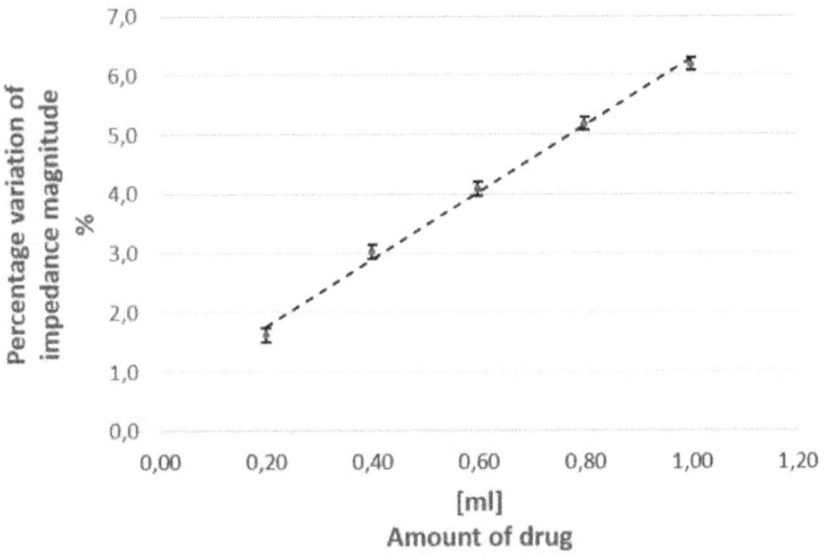

FIGURE 2.5
Impedance magnitude percentage variation according to drug amount in laboratory experiments [2].

2.5.6 Resolution

The resolution represents the smallest change in a quantity being measured that causes a perceptible change in the corresponding indication [152]. It might depend on, for example, noise (internal or external) or friction. It may also depend on the value of a quantity being measured.

In this context, the resolution is computed as the indeterminacy in the minimum measurable amount of drug, in terms of the uncertainty of the linear regression model. In particular, by mean of ANOVA, the mean squared error of the single value is estimated. In the above example of experiment, the first row of Tab. 2.1 summarizes the metrological characteristics of the presented method in order to assess the amount of drug penetrating the skin during aesthetic treatments.

2.6 Optimization

The principal parameters that affect the experimental results are investigated with the purpose to improve the sensitivity of the method, but maintaining

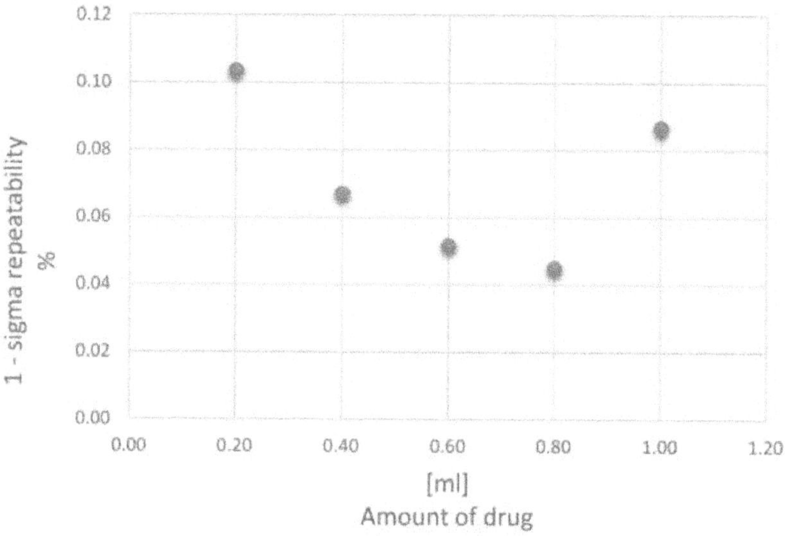

FIGURE 2.6
1-σ repeatability vs the amount of injected drug [2].

satisfying levels or resolution, repeatability, and nonlinearity. Generally, a process to be optimized has several control factors, which directly affect the target or the desired value of the output deterministically. The optimization, then, involves determining the best values, so that the output is kept at the target. It is worth noting that the words "factors" and "parameters" are synonymous; usually, engineers prefer to speak of parameters, while statisticians prefer factors instead.

2.6.1 Statistical Parameter Design

One of the most relevant problems in the engineers professional life is the quantitative experimental definition of the behaviour of a physical phenomenon, e.g., the experimental analysis of a complex device performance. The more complicated the phenomenon, the fewer analytical models of adequate approximation are available for its quantitative description. Nor is it possible to make reasonable assumptions (such as, for example, that the model of interest is simply linear). As an example, let's consider a complex device obtained by integrating several subsystems: in this case, a sufficiently precise performance model is not available and an experimental campaign must be carried out. Therefore, by means of a sequence of experiments, the relationship f which links a response η of a physical system and some experimental quantities

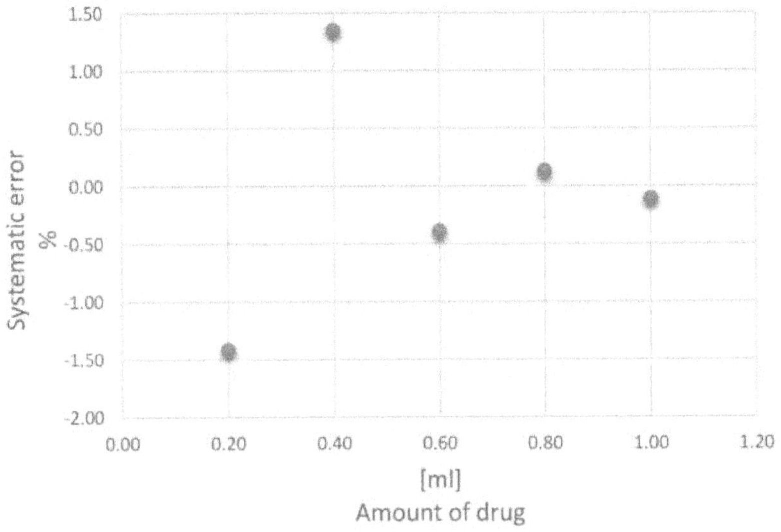

FIGURE 2.7
Percentage deterministic error considering the amount of injected drug [2].

$c_1, c_2, \ldots, c_n$ may be inferred.

$$\eta = f(c_1, c_2, \ldots, c_n). \tag{2.1}$$

For the sake of the simplicity, let's consider a modulator with a quality characteristic η, such as the modulation index, changing with the variation of some design parameters of the electronic circuit, (e.g., the values of resistors and capacitors). Otherwise, let's think to the performance of a switching power supply, where the capacity of the input capacitor is to be varied to stabilize the operation of the converter; or the parameters of the output filter and the power levels.

In statistics, the *Response Surface Method* (RSM) [155] allows to quantitatively and efficiently explore the relationships between different explanatory quantities (parameters or factors) and one or more response quantities (quality characteristic). The method was introduced by George E. P. Box and K. B. Wilson in 1951. It finds, at least, three very important applications in engineering:

- modelling of a prototype characteristics;
- metrological characterization;
- parameter optimization.

The main idea of the RSM method is to use a sequence of experiments duly designed to infer the experimental law of the quality characteristic behaviour according to the parameters variation. Box and Wilson, in particular, suggest the use of a polynomial model taking into account the superposition and interactions of the parameters. They recognize that this model is only an approximation, since it is easy to estimate and apply, even with a poor knowledge about the process. However, contrary to conventional methods, the interaction between the process quantities can be determined by means of statistical techniques. Statistical approaches, such as RSM, can also be employed to maximize the production of a special substance by optimizing operational factors (experimental techniques of parametric optimization, Statistical Parameter Design) [3].

In defining a campaign of experiments, sufficient resources in terms of time and money are not always available to acquire all the necessary information on a certain physical phenomenon. Actually, in practice there are constraints on the cost and timing of the experimental investigation, so maximum information is to be taken with the minimum number of measurements. Therefore, one of the most common problems in the field of measurements consists precisely in optimizing the experimental effort with the accuracy of the resulted information.

The Design Of the Experiments provides a scientific answer to this problem [156]. It allows to define the minimum number of experiments necessary to obtain a predetermined precision in the identification and experimental validation of the theoretical model of the phenomenon under consideration. The main criterion takes only the information necessary for the particular model hypothesized, by verifying its significance a posteriori. A simple example can illustrate this criterion. To determine the coefficients of a one-dimensional linear model: (*i*) the experiments are carried out only in three points, (*ii*) the values of the coefficients are identified by means of a least squares analysis, (*iii*) the hypothesis of linearity is verified a posteriori, and (*iv*) the quality of the coefficient is estimated by means of a one-way ANOVA analysis.

In general, an easy way to estimate a polynomial model is to use a factorial experiment or a fractional factorial design. This is sufficient to determine which explanatory quantities affect the response of interest. Once it is suspected that only significant explanatory quantities are left, a more complicated design can be implemented, such as a central composite design to estimate a second degree polynomial model, which is still only an approximation. However, the second-degree model can be used to optimize (maximize, minimize, or achieve a specific goal) the response quantities of interest.

In the following, the basic concepts of the Design of the Experiments ("Definitions") are initially presented, by making an in-depth study on modelling ("The model"), as well as some useful statistical tests. Subsequently, the fundamental techniques for using the "Complete Factorial Experiments" are illustrated. The "Fractional Factorial Experiments" are then described because they allow to reduce the experimental effort with the same information content. In particular, the "Plans with multiple Multilevel Factors" are examined. The theoretical foundations, as well as more details on the various possible experimental schemes, are beyond the scope of this exposition and can easily be found in the specialized texts [3, 155–157].

2.6.2 Design of Experiments

Let's assume to have to collect experimental information on a characteristic quality of a system influenced by several controllable parameters (factors) whose values (levels) can vary in certain intervals. The set of values that all the parameters can assume, once their range has been limited, is called experimental space. In their range of variability, the parameters can be discrete or continuous. Actually, the number of levels, even if high, is however limited by the physical resolution of the measure. Moreover, in practice a finite number of "samples", also for continuous parameters, is identified in order to reduce the number of experiments. Consequently, the experimental space becomes a limited and discrete domain, whose number of distinct points n_p is defined according to combinatorial analysis as:

$$n_p = \prod_i (n_{li})^{n_{fi}} \tag{2.2}$$

where n_{fi} indicates the number of the i-th group of factors having n_{li} levels.

In many circumstances, the value of n_p can be very high and thus, the problem of obtaining the maximum information with the minimum experimental effort arises.

In this case, it is advisable to carry out a factorial experiment (or experiment plan): the data are collected from a sequence of tests where the levels of a parameter are changed appropriately. This allows to systematically explore the experimental space following a logic that optimizes the experimental effort, according to the objective of the investigation.

In each test, the factor levels are set in such a way that the system assumes a certain configuration. The test is performed through a predefined protocol to keep constant the experimental conditions. All the parameters that affect the system under test, the measurement system and the environment are determined in order to make the experiment repeatable.

A first approach to factorial experimentation, typical of common logic, considers only some configurations corresponding to particular levels of factors, measuring the quality characteristic only in specific points of the experimental space. Such particular levels are chosen on the basis of considerations related to their significance of the specific problem under examination, or in general equally spaced in the experimental space. Very often they are assumed according to an arbitrary logic, dictated by criteria of comfort in experimentation. On the other hand, according to a more rigorous approach, the combination of the levels of factors to be used in each experiment must be chosen on the basis of criteria aimed at the objectives of the experimental investigation. Neglecting them can, in fact, cause incorrect estimates of the effects of the factors on the quality characteristic and/or incorrect estimates of the experimental error and, therefore, incorrect deductions.

2.6.2.1 Fractional Factorial Experiments

When higher-order effects, such as quadratic or cubic effects, are to be evaluated, the factors with more than two levels must be included in the experiments.

In industrial practice it is customary to consider three-level factors to evaluate at least the sign of the curvature of the quality characteristic. This is of extreme practical importance as it allows to evaluate the optimum point.

The Japanese quality engineer Genichi Taguchi has developed a family of orthogonal planes (Taguchi orthogonal arrays) with suitably restricted randomization [3,155]. They have a considerable practical utility: the columns are organized in such a way that the number of level changes increases from left to right in the matrix (Fig. 2.8). This allows the experimenter to immediately assign to the leftmost columns the factors characterized by greater practical difficulty in changing their levels.

The Fig. 2.8 shows some examples of Taguchi orthogonal matrices. They are denoted with the symbol $L_j(i^k)$ indicating the number of rows and columns, as well as the number of levels in each column. For example, the matrix L9 (3^4), has 9 rows, 4 columns, each with 3 levels; while L18 $(2^1, 3^7)$, has 18 rows, 1 column with two levels, and 7 with 3 levels.

2.6.3 Setup Optimization

The parameters considered here are the drug conductivity, the electrodes surface and gap, and the signal frequency and amplitude. The influence of these parameters on the metrological characteristics is investigated by means of a statistical parameter design, based on a Taguchi experimental plan L18 [157]. This plan represents a well organized set of experiments where all the parameters of interest are varied over a specified range, where 18 is the number of experimental runs.

Among the selected parameters, the electrodes surface and gaps are directly linked to the dimension of the investigation volume, and the location of the maximum concentration of current flowing through the sample under test. Likewise, the drug conductivity and the signal amplitude are directly related to the measurement sensitivity. Meanwhile, considering the contribution of the injected drug predominantly ohmic, the signal frequency should be characterized by an inverse relationship with the sensitivity.

About the electrodes dimensions, three different electrodes surface levels are identified as fraction of the original electrode surface of 7.28 cm^2: 1.00, 0.50, 0.25, in order to simplify their cut. Then, by evaluating the sample size,

Run	Columns		
	1	2	3
1	1	1	1
2	1	2	2
3	2	1	2
4	2	2	1

L4(2³)

Run	Columns						
	1	2	3	4	5	6	7
1	1	1	1	1	1	1	1
2	1	1	1	2	2	2	2
3	1	2	2	1	1	2	2
4	1	2	2	2	2	1	1
5	2	1	2	1	2	1	2
6	2	1	2	2	1	2	1
7	2	2	1	1	2	2	1
8	2	2	1	2	1	1	2

L8(2⁷)

Run	Columns			
	1	2	3	4
1	1	1	1	1
2	1	2	2	2
3	1	3	3	3
4	2	1	2	3
5	2	2	3	1
6	2	3	1	2
7	3	1	3	2
8	3	2	1	3
9	3	3	2	1

L9(3⁴)

Run	Columns							
	1	2	3	4	5	6	7	8
1	1	1	1	1	1	1	1	1
2	1	1	2	2	2	2	2	2
3	1	1	3	3	3	3	3	3
4	1	2	1	1	2	2	3	3
5	1	2	2	2	3	3	1	1
6	1	2	3	3	1	1	2	2
7	1	3	1	2	1	3	2	3
8	1	3	2	3	2	1	3	1
9	1	3	3	1	3	2	1	2
10	2	1	1	3	3	2	2	1
11	2	1	2	1	1	3	3	2
12	2	1	3	2	2	1	1	3
13	2	2	1	2	3	1	3	2
14	2	2	2	3	1	2	1	3
15	2	2	3	1	2	3	2	1
16	2	3	1	3	2	3	1	2
17	2	3	2	1	3	1	2	3
18	2	3	3	2	1	2	3	1

L18(2¹3⁷)

Run	Columns												
	1	2	3	4	5	6	7	8	9	10	11	12	13
1	1	1	1	1	1	1	1	1	1	1	1	1	1
2	1	1	1	1	2	2	2	2	2	2	2	2	2
3	1	1	1	1	3	3	3	3	3	3	3	3	3
4	1	2	2	2	1	1	1	2	2	2	3	3	3
5	1	2	2	2	2	2	2	3	3	3	1	1	1
6	1	2	2	2	3	3	3	1	1	1	2	2	2
7	1	3	3	3	1	1	1	3	3	3	2	2	2
8	1	3	3	3	2	2	2	1	1	1	3	3	3
9	1	3	3	3	3	3	3	2	2	2	1	1	1
10	2	1	2	3	1	2	3	1	2	3	1	2	3
11	2	1	2	3	2	3	1	2	3	1	2	3	1
12	2	1	2	3	3	1	2	3	1	2	3	1	2
13	2	2	3	1	1	2	3	2	3	1	3	1	2
14	2	2	3	1	2	3	1	3	1	2	1	2	3
15	2	2	3	1	3	1	2	1	2	3	2	3	1
16	2	3	1	2	1	2	3	3	1	2	2	3	1
17	2	3	1	2	2	3	1	1	2	3	3	1	2
18	2	3	1	2	3	1	2	2	3	1	1	2	3
19	3	1	3	2	1	3	2	1	3	2	1	3	2
20	3	1	3	2	2	1	3	2	1	3	2	1	3
21	3	1	3	2	3	2	1	3	2	1	3	2	1
22	3	2	1	3	1	3	2	2	1	3	3	2	1
23	3	2	1	3	2	1	3	3	2	1	1	3	2
24	3	2	1	3	3	2	1	1	3	2	2	1	3
25	3	3	2	1	1	3	2	3	2	1	2	1	3
26	3	3	2	1	2	1	3	1	3	2	3	2	1
27	3	3	2	1	3	2	1	2	1	3	1	3	2

L27(3¹³)

FIGURE 2.8
Examples of Taguchi orthogonal matrices: $L_j(i^k)$, j number of experiments, i number of levels, and k number of parameters with i levels [3].

when two electrodes of maximum dimensions are used, the maximum distance among them on the eggplants surface is identified equal to 4.60 cm. This value arises from the difference between the length of the specimen (10 cm) and the sum of the lengths of the two electrodes (27 mm × 2 mm). The other two further experimentation values, required to allow the infiltration of the drug, are obtained by 1.60 cm step down to a minimum of 1.40 cm.

The amplitude levels and the frequency of the stimulus signal are selected among the range provided by the commercially available instruments used for the experimental setup, i.e., the LCR Meter Agilent 4263B [151]. In particular, the frequency range varies from 0.1 kHz to 10 kHz, while the signal amplitude from 0.020 V to 1.00 V.

For the last parameter, namely the drug conductivity, a commercial drug, electrically comparable to drugs traditionally used in aesthetic medicine, such as hyaluronic acid, is exploited. This solution is used to test a conductivity variation of about 25 % (from 526 μS/cm to 666 μS/cm).

Finally, to perform the L18 plan, 18 rectangular-shaped eggplants, cut in blocks of 40 mm × 40 mm × 100 mm, are used. For each sample, the same preparation time between peeling, electrodes application and measurement, is observed. Preliminary the impedance is measured without any injected drug, then, the drug is injected in 5 consecutive steps, with the following amount: 0.2 ml, 0.4 ml, 0.6 ml, 0.8 ml, 1.0 ml, 2 cm below the eggplant surface. After each injection, the measurements are carried out by the Agilent 4263B LCR Meter.

In the *i*-th experiment of the plan L18, the measurement setup is configured according to the combination of parameters levels corresponding to the *i*-th matrix row [156], such as pointed out in Tab. 2.2.

In each experiment, the percentage variation from the initial impedance magnitude is computed for all the injected drug volumes. Each experiment is repeated 60 times, 10 for each of the 6 levels of injected drug. Then, all the metrological characteristic, and their average on 18 experiments, are computed, such as reported in the Tab. 2.2. In particular, in this table, the following parameters are listed: sensitivity [ml^{-1}], repeatability [%], nonlinearity [%], and resolution [ml].

The influence of the experiment parameters on the method sensitivity, assessed by the Analysis of Mean (ANOM) [155], is highlighted in Fig. 2.10. The ANOM is aimed at determining the effects of a certain number of parameters on a quality characteristic when more experiments are performed to reduce uncertainty.

Whereas, the statistical significance of the incidence of each parameter on the measurement sensitivity is computed by the Analysis of Variance (ANOVA). It allows to analyze the variability of the measurement results, by attributing the cause to the variation of one or more parameters, and/or to a pure random occurrence.

In the practice, the measured quantities depends on:

- the deterministic variation within a predetermined amplitude interval of one or more parameters (for example, to experimentally verify whether or not a quality characteristic is influenced by certain parameters);
- the random variation within the uncertainty range of one or more parameters (for example, to experimentally verify whether or not the uncertainty of a quantity depends on the uncertainty of some parameters).

Both the cases are analyzed using the same technique of decomposition of the variance into variance imposed by (*i*) the variation of the parameters (whether deterministic or random) and (*ii*) the variance imposed by other random sources external to the analysis.

The experimental method is, however, different in the two cases. In the first case, an interval of variation is imposed on each parameter and then, the corresponding variation imposed on the quality characteristic is determined. In the second case, it is necessary to have in the laboratory the possibility of setting the parameter values with an uncertainty much lower than the actual operating conditions. In this way, a parameters a variation equal to their uncertainty range can be imposed in order to study the effect on the uncertainty of the measured quantity.

In both the cases, it is necessary to discriminate whether the measured variability is due to a random occurrence, or actually due to the variability of

TABLE 2.2
L18 plan for statistical parameter design in performance optimization of the assessment method.

	Parameter					Results				
Run	Drug Conductivity [μS/cm]	Signal Frequency [kHz]	Electrodes Area [cm^2]	Electrodes Gap [cm]	Signal Amplitude [V]	Sensitivity [ml^{-1}]	Repeatability [%]	Nonlinearity [%]	Resolution [ml]
1	526	0.1	1.82	1.4	0.020	5.6	2.99	2.34	0.130
2	526	0.1	3.64	3.0	0.100	4.7	0.05	0.78	0.036
3	526	0.1	7 .28	4.6	1.000	3.0	0.16	3.74	0.115
4	526	1.0	1.82	1.4	0.100	4.7	1.02	4.26	0.197
5	526	1.0	3.64	3.0	1 .000	4.3	0.34	3.16	0.140
6	526	1.0	7 .28	4.6	0.020	3.1	0.03	3.69	0.118
7	526	10.0	1.82	3.0	0.020	4.3	0.89	2.54	0.107
8	526	10.0	3.64	4.6	0.100	2.7	0.32	3.80	0.098
9	526	10.0	7 .28	1.4	1 .000	2.9	0.05	2.82	0.083
10	666	0.1	1.82	4.6	1.000	4.0	0.80	1.37	0.055
11	666	0.1	3.64	1.4	0.020	4.4	0.82	1.50	0.067
12	666	0.1	7 .28	3.0	0.100	2.4	0.09	7.62	0.190
13	666	1.0	1.82	3.0	1.000	6.0	3.25	0.82	0.049
14	666	1.0	3.64	4.6	0.020	3.8	0.54	0.47	0.018
15	666	1.0	7 .28	1.4	0.100	6.4	0.95	2.26	0.113
16	666	10.0	1.82	4.6	0.100	3.6	0.61	1.00	0.036
17	666	10.0	3.64	1.4	1 .000	6.7	2.15	0.94	0.062
18	666	10.0	7 .28	3.0	0.020	2.5	0.10	2.79	0.073
					Overall mean	4.2	0.84	2.55	0.09

the parameters. This is usually discriminating by using a hypothesis testing procedure (Fisher's test) [155].

The ANOVA procedure differs depending on whether it is required to assess the global effect of all the parameters, discriminating only between the variance imposed by the parameters and the random variance, or conversely the effect of each single parameter.

The variance ratio Fi, mostly known as F-statistic [155], is computed as the ratio between the sensitivity variance due to the i-th parameter and the error variance. The histogram (Fig. 2.9), namely Pareto diagram [155], points out that the electrode gap is the most influencing parameter, followed in order by the electrode area, signal frequency, drug conductivity, and signal amplitude.

The optimum configuration, obtained by maximizing the sensitivity and with reference to the histogram of Fig. 2.10, is predicted by means of the design parameter; in particular, the optimum values of the parameters are: drug conductivity 666 μS/cm, signal frequency 1.0 kHz, electrodes area 1.82 cm^2, electrodes gap 1.4 cm, and signal amplitude 1.0 V.

It is worth to note that an increase by about 25 % in drug conductivity produces a corresponding sensitivity improvement of about 12 %.

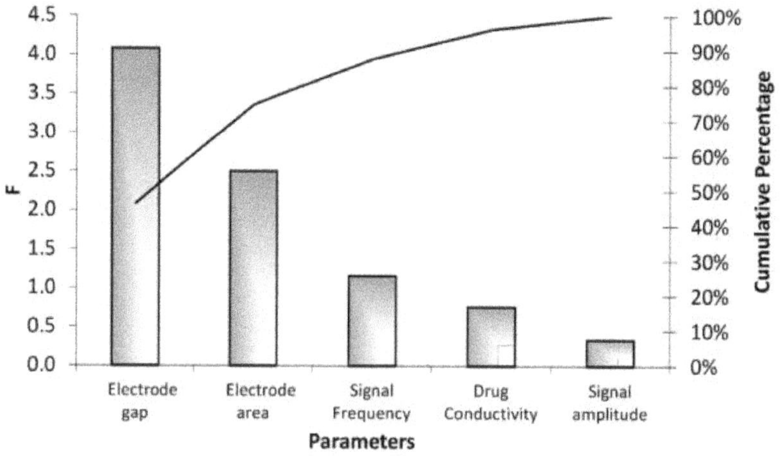

FIGURE 2.9
Ranking of parameters influence on the sensitivity [2].

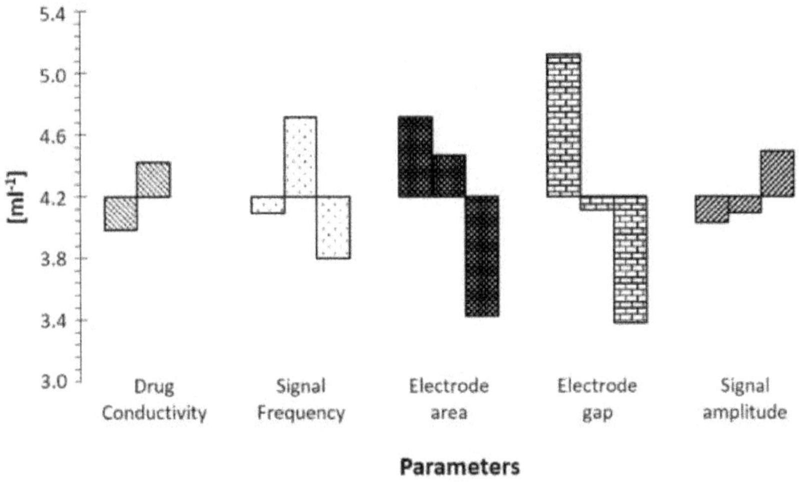

FIGURE 2.10
Influence of the experiment parameters on the method sensitivity [2].

2.7 Ex-vivo Metrological Characterization

Some of the commonly used methods for safety and efficacy testing of drugs used in aesthetic medicine include ex-vivo experiments. For the ex-vivo experiments, the living tissues are not created artificially, but directly taken from a living organism.

In the case of the above experiment, the pig skin was selected as tissue under test: according to the literature [158, 159], it is the most suitable model for human skin. Albeit ex-vivo pig skin is closer to in-vivo conditions, it is, however, less reactive biologically to a treatment or a stress.

Ex-vivo models can be more accurate in representing human skin, particularly to investigate the transdermal delivery of an ingredient or drug after topical application. In fact, several properties of porcine and human skins, such as epidermal thickness and lipid composition, as well as the permeability of the membranes to diverse compounds, are significantly similar [160].

For the ex-vivo experiments described here, three ears of domestic pigs are used, bought by a local abattoir, with less than few post-mortem hours. The experiment is then immediately conducted in a laboratory environment, with minimal alteration of the organisms natural conditions. Dead cells of the stratum corneum are removed by applying a 5 cm × 5 cm tape, and detached with a single movement for 20 times.

The setup configuration is the same as used in the in-vitro experiments, including the solution. The only difference is the drug injection depth, reduced to 0.5 cm.

Analogously as for the laboratory experiments, a linear trend is experienced (Fig. 2.11). In Tab. 2.3, the obtained metrological characteristics of ex-vivo tests are compared with laboratory performance in the same conditions. It follows that:

- the sensitivity increases significantly, due to the reduced injection depth;
- a higher nonlinearity is detected, namely 5.04 % compared to 3.64 %;
- the 1-σ repeatability decreases from 0.11 % to 0.47 %, owing to the higher variability in electrical response of death pig cells with respect to eggplant;
- the accuracy decreases from 4.38 % to 6.20 %, owing to the lower average reproducibility intrinsic to ex-vivo experiments;
- the resolution worsens from 0.35 ml to 0.44 ml.

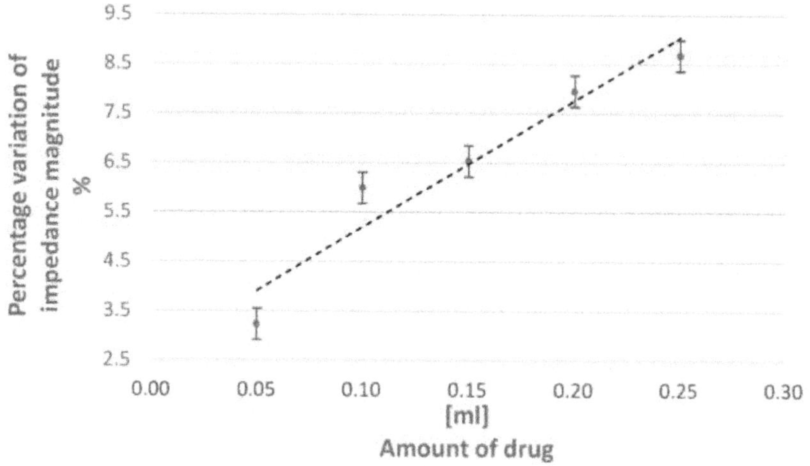

FIGURE 2.11
Impedance magnitude percentage variation vs drug amount in ex-vivo experiments [2].

TABLE 2.3
Metrological characteristics of the impedance-based method for assessing the injected drug.

	Sensitivity $[ml^{-1}]$	Nonlinearity [%]	1-σ Repeatability [%]	Accuracy [%]	Resolution [ml]
Laboratory exp.	30.6	3.64	0.11	4.38	0.35
Ex-vivo exp.	34.4	5.04	0.47	6.20	0.44

3

Hyaluronic Acid Meter

CONTENTS

The whole process of developing an on-chip instrument, the Drug Under Skin Meter (DUSM), is illustrated for aesthetic applications. The DUSM assess the amount of an aesthetic drug (e.g., hyaluronic acid) penetrated after transdermal delivery, by measuring tissue impedance variation before and after the delivery. The design of the instrument is described by focusing on the architecture and the operating characteristics. The metrological characterization under controlled laboratory conditions is reported. Then, the calibration procedure, using reference passive electronic components, is outlined. Significant results for clinical applications are reported in terms of uncertainty, and they are consistent with the metrological targets of the DUSM design.

3.1 Design

The Drug Under Skin Meter (DUSM), an on-chip instrument, monitors the amount of drug actually penetrated into the tissue, after a transdermal treatment, by assessing the difference between the impedance magnitude before and after the administration. Below, the *Architecture* and the *Operation* of the instrument are reported.

DOI: 10.1201/9781003170143-3

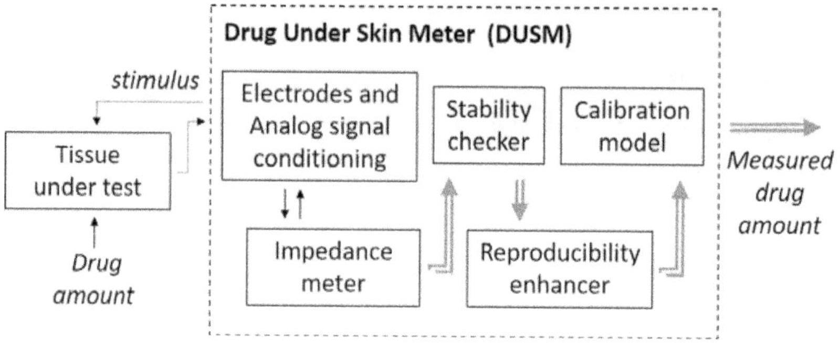

FIGURE 3.1
Architecture of the DUSM [4].

3.1.1 Architecture

The block diagram of the DUSM is depicted in Fig. 3.1. The *Tissue under test* can be a whatever biological tissue, ranging from eggplants to pig skin and to human skin. In the tissue under test, a known amount of drug is injected. The *Electrodes and Analog Signal Conditioning* block stimulates the tissue under test by a sinusoidal current at a given frequency. The corresponding voltage drop is acquired through pre-gelled electrodes. Then, after the analog-to-digital conversion, the impedance magnitude is computed by the *Impedance meter.*

During the measurement, the electrode gel progressively penetrates the tissue and impacts on its conductivity [21,153]. Therefore, a stability loss arises. Before the drug delivery, the *Stability checker* measures the tissue impedance. Then, it analyzes the time trend of the drift to proper compensate this phenomenon.

Different tissues exhibit peculiar electrical behaviours. The *Reproducibility enhancer* uses a normalization factor to attenuate the effects of the variability of skin electrical reaction to drug delivery. To this aim, the initial measurements are averaged and a specific value for each tissue under test is identified before drug administration. Then, the successive measurements are normalized to this specific value. In this way, the impact of the initial conditions and the common mode noise are soften.

After the drug administration, a *Calibration model* calculates the amount of drug actually under the tissue through an experimentally identified model. The model receives the normalized impedance variation in input. Finally, on this basis, the model assesses the amount of drug penetrating into the tissue.

3.1.2 Operation

The DUSM works according to the following steps:

- *Tissue preparation*: generally, the tissue must be appropriately treated before the measurement. In particular, the surface of the stratum corneum has to be removed in order to increase the stability of electrodes-skin contact. Moreover, the thinning of the stratum corneum is useful to decrease the negative impact of its impedance on the measurement sensitivity. The corneum abrasion can be carried out by an acetone gauze, an abrasive film, or an adhesive tape. Nevertheless, the residual stratum corneum still represents a relevant uncertainty source. Furthermore, the sebum is removed to reduce the measurement uncertainty related to the pH of the skin;

- *Electrode application*: during the measurement, a good electrodes-skin contact must be guaranteed, even in case of movements of the patient. Therefore, pre-gelled electrodes are exploited due to their good adhesion strength. The used gel is a conductive and biocompatible material; it is made up of NaOH (sodium-hydroxide), which acts as a neutralizing agent, NaCl (Sodium chloride), Carbomer, as a thickening agent, EDTA (Ethylenediaminetetraacetic acid tetrasodium salt, dihydrate) as a complexing agent, and deionized H_2O (water deprived by hydrogen and hydroxide ions of dissolved minerals) and demineralized (i.e., free of mineral salts and limestone);

- *Drift monitoring*: after the electrodes are applied, the tissue impedance is monitored for 10 s. At a frequency of 1 kHz, the drift due to the gel penetration is assessed and compensated;

- *Tissue identification*: the average of the impedance values measured for 10 s by the *Stability checker* is calculated. All the successive impedance variations are normalized by the same initial average value;

- *Measurement of the conveyed drug amount*: the tissue impedance is measured at the frequency of 1 kHz after transdermal drug administration. The relationship between the normalized impedance variation and the drug amount actually penetrated is well described by a linear model. This model, obtained from the previous calibration, accepts the measured normalized impedance variation at the input and produces the amount of drug at the output [2].

3.2 Realization

Off-the-shelf components are exploited for the DUSM realization [161]. Therefore, the cost of procurement and development results very low, and also the maintenance is almost cheap. As shown in Fig. 3.2 (a), the DUSM is connected to pre-gelled electrodes in a framework of in-vivo clinical trial. Power is supplied from a laptop via a USB cable. Moreover, Fig. 3.2 (b) shows the motherboard provided as evaluation kit [162] from Analog Device.

(a)

(b)

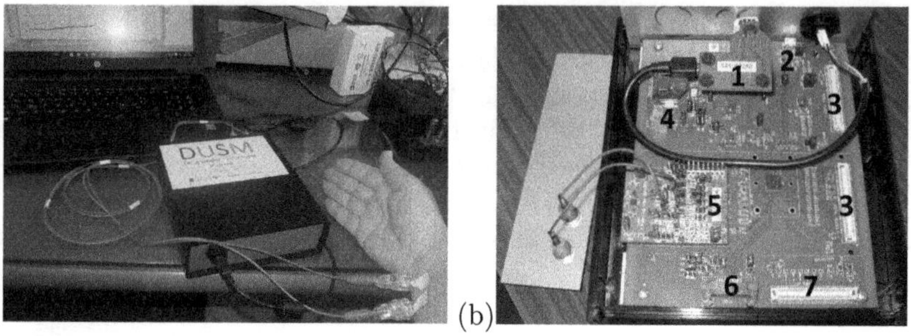

FIGURE 3.2
The realized instrument: (a) operation view and (b) motherboard (1: Universal Asynchronous Receiver-Transmitter, 2: USB, 3: peripheral connector, 4: external power supply, 5: analog signal conditioning, 6: firmware monitoring connector, and 7: cap-touch connector) [4].

3.2.1 Hardware

The DUSM is a low-cost, portable, and flexible device, suitable to perform accurate bioimpedance measurements. Its core is represented by the board ADuCM350 by Analog Device. The ADuCM350 is a complete, coin-cell powered, high-precision, on-chip meter for generic portable applications. Its applications include point-of-care diagnostics and body-worn devices for monitoring vital signs. The ADuCM350 with a 16 MHz processor ARM Cortex-M3, equipped with an analog front-end, is specifically designed for high-precision amperometric, voltmetric, and impedimetric measurements. Therefore, this specific board is implemented inside the DUSM as an impedance meter.

In the following, a short description of the main functional blocks of the device is presented.

- A precision ac voltage source
  The configuration, shown in Fig. 3.3, is based on a closed-loop block, in order to give a precision ac voltage to the sensor. This block includes a 12-bit digital-to-analog converter (DAC). Meanwhile, a low-pass RC filter (50 kHz) is used to reduce the noise of the generated signal, and a programmable gain amplifier (PGA) is used to pre-amplify the filtered signal. Then, the signal is given to the excitation amplifier loop. In this way, a voltage, precise enough for the present application, is generated at the selected frequency;

- A high-precision current meter
  As shown in Fig. 3.4, the board adopts a transimpedance amplifier (TIA), since the currents flowing in the measured impedance are usually in the range of micro- or nano-ampere. The TIA is realized with an operational amplifier in inverted configuration, with a bias voltage V_{BIAS} on a common-mode voltage of 1.1 V, using an external resistor R_{TIA}, whose value defines the

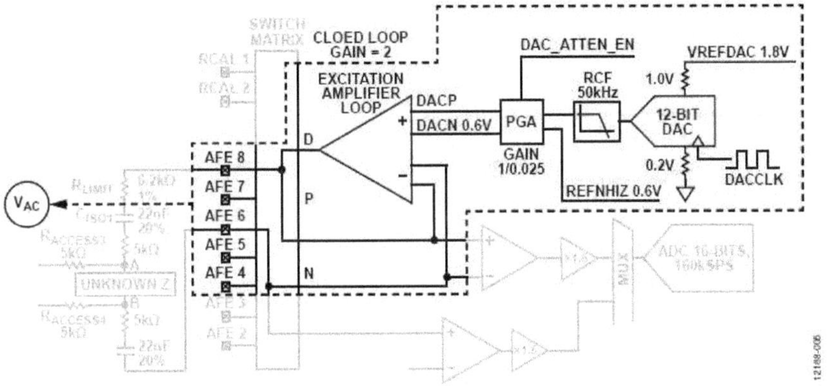

FIGURE 3.3
AC voltage source on ADuCM350 (in light grey the other blocks of the ADuCM350) [5].

gain. In this way, a voltage can be measured by using an analog-to-digital converter (ADC). The ADC converts the signal at a sampling rate of 160 kSa/s with 16 bits of quantization. Moreover, a Discrete Fourier Transform is carried out on 2048 samples, and the resulting real and imaginary components for the current measurements are calculated;

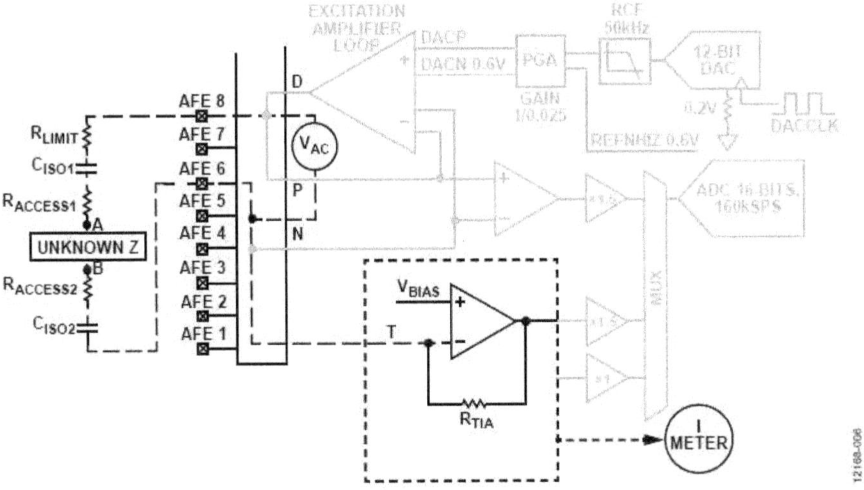

FIGURE 3.4
High precision current meter (in light grey the other blocks of the ADuCM350) [5].

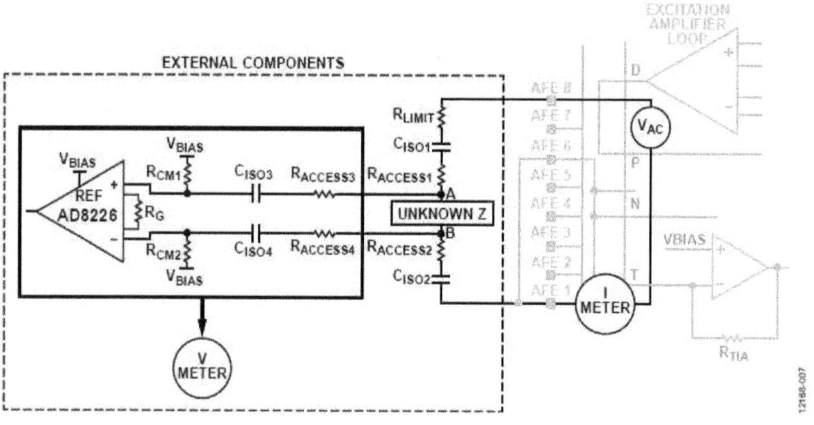

FIGURE 3.5
High precision differential voltage meter [5].

- A precision differential voltage meter
  Another section of the board is presented in Fig. 3.5. The voltage drop, across the unknown measurand, is sensed by means of a low-power amplifier with high signal-to-noise ratio and common-mode rejection (AD8226). This operation amplifier is referenced off the common mode of the system, set by the V_{BIAS} voltage on the TIA channel. Through one of the auxiliary channels (AN_A) of ADuCM350, the output of the operational amplifier is acquired. Then, the ADC converts the auxiliary voltage measurement with a sampling frequency of 160 kSa/s. A 2048-point DFT is performed on the data, in order to assess the real and imaginary components of the voltage.

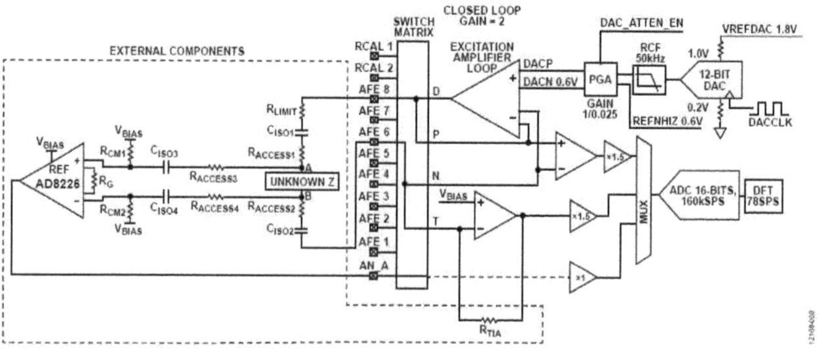

FIGURE 3.6
Block diagram of measurement system the on-chip impedance spectroscope ADuCM350 [5].

All the above mentioned sections are sketched in Fig. 3.6, which shows the entire measurement scheme. Once obtained the current and the voltage DFT measurements, the device can assess the measured impedance using the following equations,

$$\begin{gathered}
Voltage\ Measurement\ Magnitude = \sqrt{(r_v^2 + i_v^2)} \\
Voltage\ Measurement\ Phase = Atan(\tfrac{i_v}{r_v}) \\
Current\ Measurement\ Magnitude = \sqrt{(r_c^2 + i_c^2)} \\
Current\ Measurement\ Phase = Atan(\tfrac{i_c}{r_c})
\end{gathered} \tag{3.1}$$

where r and i are the real and imaginary components of the voltage and the current DFT measurements, respectively. The unknown impedance Z_x is assessed by applying the Ohm's law, where the ratio between voltage and current magnitudes takes into account also the gains of the signal chains as follows:

$$Z(Magnitude) = \left(\frac{Voltage\ Magnitude}{Current\ Magnitude}\right) * \left(\frac{1.5}{1.494}\right) * R_{TIA} \tag{3.2}$$

The current value is converted to a voltage, using the R_{TIA}, for measurement purposes. The gain must be taken into account. The gain value of 1.5 in the previous equation is the ratio between the gain of the current measurement channel (which is 1.5) vs the gain of the voltage measurement channel (which is 1.0).

The selection of the value R_G allows to determine the input amplifier gain; for the AD8226 it is assessed by the following relation:

$$R_G = \frac{(49.4\ k\Omega)}{(G-1)}. \tag{3.3}$$

By choosing R_G=100 kΩ, the resulting gain is 1.494.

It is necessary to guarantee the safety of both patients and operator when medical electrical equipment is involved, that can potentially be hazardous if not properly managed. Hence, it is indispensable that the voltage and the amplitude values of the injected current meet safety requirements, such as those prescribed by IEC-60601 [147].

Compliance with IEC-60601 standard [147] is essential in the context of safe operation of medical equipment, since it provides general requirements for basic safety and essential performance requirements of all kind of medical electrical equipment.

The DUSM achieves the safety requirements by suitable analog signal conditioning, based mainly on the instrumentation amplifier AD8226 by Analog Devices. The IEC-60601 standards [147], for patient/wearer safety and effectiveness of medical electrical equipment, specifies the limits of leakage and auxiliary currents under normal and single-fault conditions. If the excitation frequency is less than or equal to 1 kHz, the limit of the maximum RMS current allowed by the international safety standards is 10 μA. The lower frequency limit is selected by considering that at frequency between 50 Hz and 1 kHz neurons are very sensitive to the current. If the excitation frequency f is greater than 1 kHz, the maximum current is defined as:

$$I_{AC_{MAX}} = \frac{f}{1000\,Hz} \cdot 10\,\mu A_{RMS} \tag{3.4}$$

DUSM uses voltage excitation in impedance measurements. A 3-kΩ protective resistor is inserted so that the current, with an applied voltage of 100 mV, does not exceed the peak value of 8 μA, well below the above limit of 10 μA. The device is powered via USB from laptop in standby, and via its own battery, during in-vivo working.

For impedance measurements, the DUSM exploits voltage excitation. In order to not exceed the current limit standard, a 3 kΩ protective resistor is inserted. This means that, to be on safe side, when a voltage of 100 mV is applied, the current cannot exceed the peak value of 8 μA, which is fair below the above-said limit of 10 μA.

Moreover, the device can be powered via USB from laptop in standby or via a rechargeable battery, which makes the system isolated from the main supply and inherently safe with reference to ac and ground leakage currents.

3.2.2 Firmware

Analog Devices provide libraries for basic operations to perform impedance measurements. On this basis, the firmware of the DUSM was developed by introducing useful functions to allow the correct operation of the instrument. In particular, the firmware design is based on the software package ADuCM350BBCZ in order to implement applications for the ADuCM350 [5]. The ADuCM350BBCZ is prototyped to work with IAR Embedded Workbench for ARM and the Micrium uC/OS-II RTOS for ARM Cortex-M3 [163]. The firmware is implemented in C. Device Drivers and System Services are adopted for on-chip peripherals configuration. During the initialization stage, power up and calibration steps are carried out. All the arithmetic is performed by a custom fixed-point type, with 28 integer bits and 4 fractional bits. The block diagram of the firmware is illustrated in Fig. 3.7.

- *Main*: it is the main block of the firmware, and is started when the device is turned on;

- *Measures Manager*: this block implements the initialization logic of all hardware and callbacks (functions recalled following an interrupt) to react to key pressure and is based on the AFE system libraries;

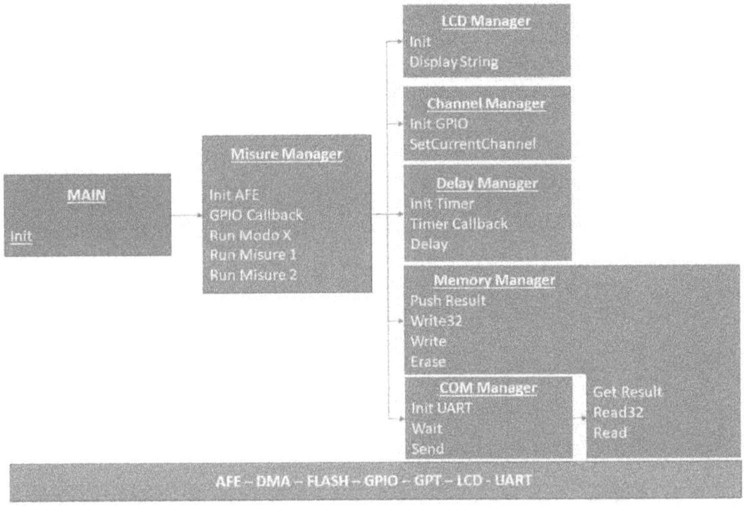

FIGURE 3.7
Block diagram of the DUSM firmware (AFE: Analog Front-End, DMA: Direct Memory Access, GPIO: General-Purpose Input/Output, GPT: GUID Partition Table, LCD: Liquid Crystal Display, UART: Universal Asynchronous Receiver-Transmitter).

- *LCD Manager*: this block includes the functions of initialization and display of the tests on the LCD display and is based on the internal GPIO and LCD libraries, useful for future upgrade of the device;
- *Channel Manager*: this block includes the functions of initialization of the processor outputs and the driving of the pins to change the channel; and it is based on the internal GPIO libraries;
- *Delay Manager*: this block implements the initialization of the internal timer and the functions for waiting, via callback, for the time needed during measurements and is based on the internal GPT libraries;
- *Memory Manager*: this block implements the logic for writing, reading and block allocation in the internal memory as well as the low-level writing functions and is based on the internal DMA and FLASH libraries;
- *COM Manager*: it contains the initialization of communication on the UART and the management logic of the communication protocol with the external software interface and is based on the internal UART libraries.

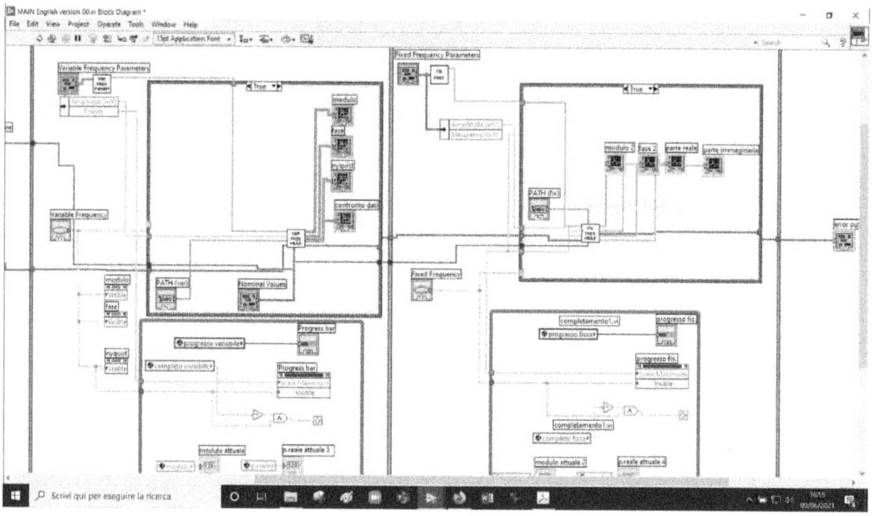

FIGURE 3.8
LabVIEW software: block diagram.

3.2.3 Software

The software of the DUSM was developed in LabVIEW® by National Instruments. In Fig. 3.8, the block diagram of developed software is shown. The following main features were considered:

- A user-friendly interface, able to assist the operator in performing the measurements during the drug transdermal delivery, as well as to assess the amount of drug absorbed by the tissue under examination;
- A system able to perform different types of measurements that allows the selection of fixed or variable frequency by the operator;
- A system able to perform the calibration on circuits with known impedance;
- An easy and fast communication with a PC (via serial communication protocol), for saving and, subsequently, processing the acquired measurement data.

A variable frequency of impedance measurement is used in the preliminary study phases, in order to obtain information on the properties of the tissue under test and its characteristics. Thus, the tissue can be classified and the parameters of the inverse model can be obtained.

On the other hand, the fixed frequency measurement, mainly used during clinical practice, is used to measure the amount of drug absorbed, hence, the bioavailability.

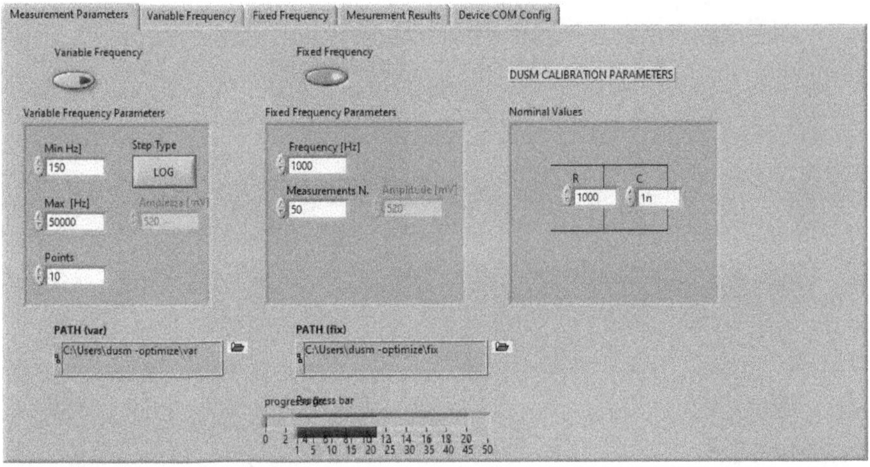

FIGURE 3.9
LabVIEW Software: Front panel.

Finally, the last implemented mode allows to carry out tests on known samples or reference standards to calibrate the instrument.

An example of the front panel of the user interface is illustrated in Fig. 3.9. The three different modes are shown, for the variable frequency the amplitude and the frequency range can be set between 150 Hz and 50 kHz, and for each frequency 10 measurements are performed. The last mode, instead, allows to set the resistor and the capacitor values. In Fig. 3.10 can be noted: in the foreground the DUSM and the personal computer, and on the background the LabVIEW software running.

3.3 Metrological Characterization

The primary goal of this section is to highlight the metrological characterization of the DUSM, on reference passive electronic components. The impedance spectroscope is tested separately, while, in the next chapters, all the measurement configurations as well as the DUSM as a whole, will be tested. Therefore, the measurement process and the instrument are evaluated in terms of the resulting uncertainty.

A measurement can be thought as a well-run production process having the measures as output. The measurement quality is the main issue, and is quantified in different ways; the main one is surely in terms of uncertainty. Without such an assessment, the results of an instrument cannot be judged, or

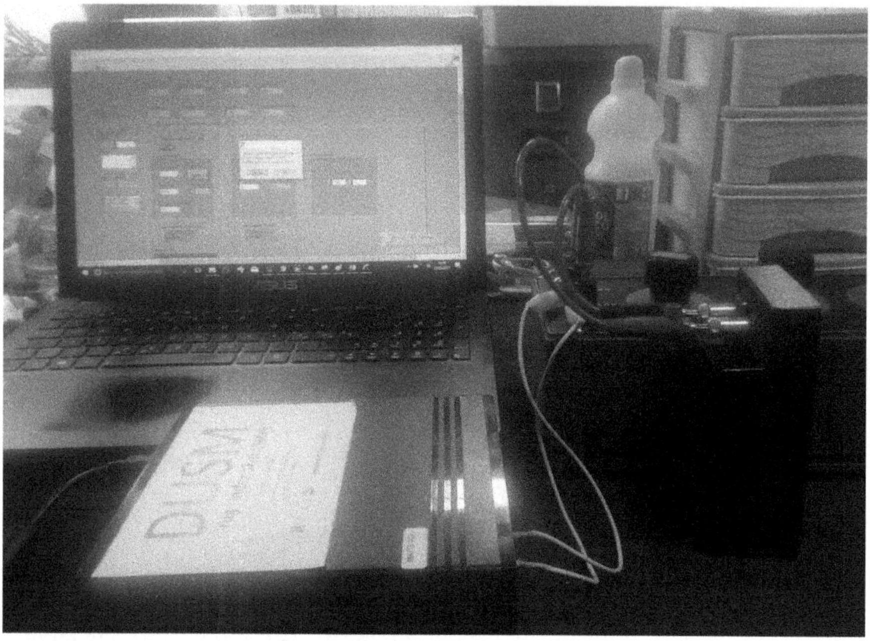

FIGURE 3.10
LabVIEW software running.

a suitable basis cannot be established for making decisions relating to health, safety, commercial, or scientific excellence.

The device is characterized by analyzing the deterministic and random undesired contributions, together with the calibration curves necessary to correct the deterministic errors.

The following subsections outline the procedures for calibration. Instrumental measurement uncertainty is obtained through the calibration, a measurement process that assigns values to the response of an instrument by referring to reference standards or a designated measurement process. Thus, the calibration procedure compares a new instrument with reference standards, according to a specific experimental set up.

In Fig. 3.11, the setup for the DUSM calibration is shown. The DUSM is connected to twofold reference standards, namely, a calibrated decade resistor ("EuroOhm" model N:85005) and a calibrated capacitor (General Radio 509-F serial no:4476).

3.3.1 Impedance Spectroscope Tests

Experimental setup

The instrument is calibrated by using different reference resistors, simple

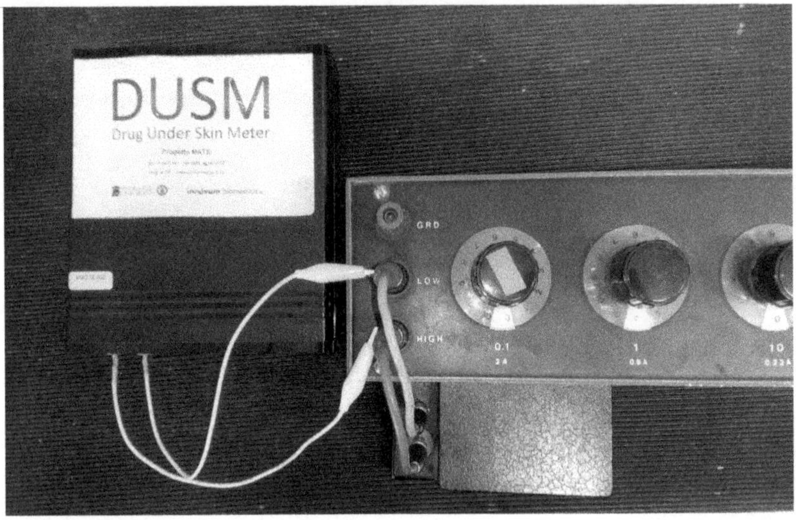

FIGURE 3.11
DUSM Calibration.

parallel RC or with series with another resistor; in particular, the reference sample, with impedance values included in the physiological range of bioimpedance. According to the typical values of skin electrical impedance [2]: a parallel of a resistance $(4500.0 \pm 0.1)\ \Omega$ and a capacitance (1.0 ± 0.1) nF is put in series with another resistance $(300.0 \pm 0.1)\ \Omega$, obtained by means of two Uniohm 85005 Decade Resistors, and the Standard Capacitor Type 509-F, by General Radio.

Calibration

It is important to have reliable and highly accurate measurements. Therefore, it is fundamental that instruments used within any measuring system have to be calibrated. Thus, a key measurement concept is calibration, which is the comparison of an instrument or device against a more accurate instrument, certified reference materials, or other reference condition, to determine the metrological performance characteristics of an instrument. Calibration establishes the reliability of the instrument, besides it ensures that readings from the instrument are consistent with other measurements, and so, it allows to determine the accuracy of the instrument readings [152].

To this aim, under repeatability conditions, that is, all measurements carried out under the same conditions, 32 measurements are carried out at a room temperature of 24 °C, using a sine wave amplitude of 100 mV. The sample mean of these 32 measurements can be modelled as a random variable with normal probability distribution. This value is specified for in-vivo working of DUSM, according to its design and due to safety reason. Meanwhile,

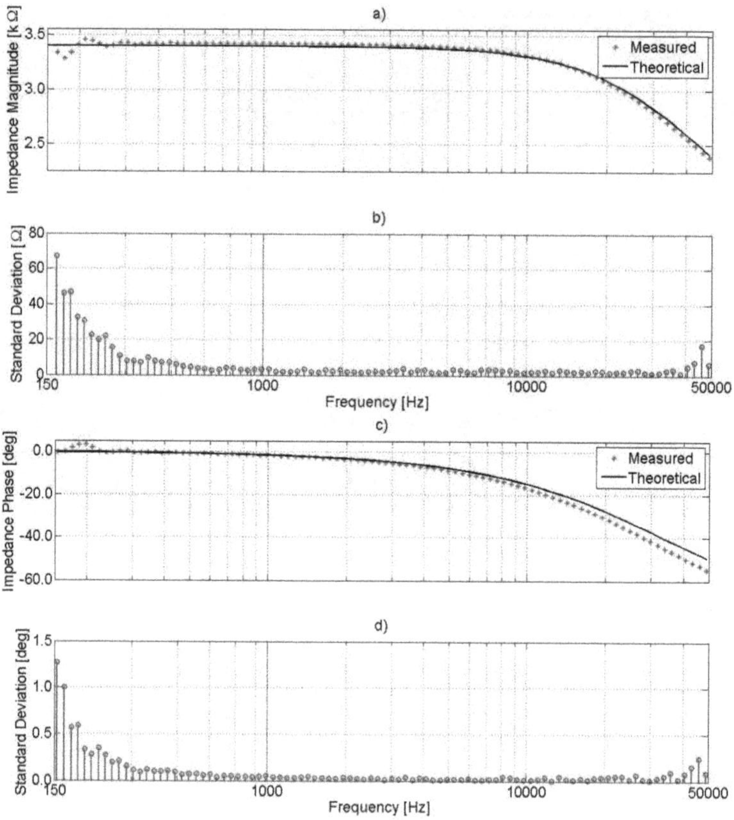

FIGURE 3.12
Calibration results of the DUSM impedance spectroscope, after offset and gain error compensation: (a) reference and measured impedance magnitude values with (b) 1-σ repeatability, and (c) reference and measured impedance phase values with (d) 1-σ repeatability [4].

the frequency varies from 150 Hz to 49 kHz through constant steps over a logarithmic scale. Then, the mean and standard deviation of impedance magnitude and phase are computed. The results are compared with the reference values obtained by the mathematical model built with an RC loop in series with a further resistor. The deterministic error is compensated together with offset and gain errors.

The results are reported in Fig. 3.12. The first plot (a) shows reference (black line) and measured (red stars) impedance magnitude values, with 1-σ repeatability reported in plot (b). Specifically, 1-σ repeatability defines a coverage interval for the measurement results, estimated by the sample mean.

This interval is defined as $[\mu - \sigma; \mu + \sigma]$ and it includes 68 % of possible measurand values when assuming a normal distribution.

The plot (c) reports reference and measured impedance phase values, with (d) 1-σ repeatability. Finally, in the bandwidth of interest, a percentage deterministic errors on the magnitude of 1 % and of 7 Ω is obtained. Whereas, the percentage deterministic error of phase is 12 %; thus, the results are consistent with the metrological targets of the DUSM design; despite the DUSM performances are not optimal at low frequency, as shown in the figure.

4

Measurement Method for Diabetology

CONTENTS

In this chapter, a measurement method for assessing insulin bioavailability in diabetology is illustrated. Firstly, an electrochemical characterization of an insulin solution is presented. Indeed, the knowledge of the insulin electrical signature allows a more accurate assessment of its impact on the impedance variation of an infiltered tissue can be assured. Specifically, the analysis is implemented at varying progressively the active principle in the insulin solution under test, in order to separate the impact of both the solute and the solvent on the impedance variation. The higher the concentration level of insulin is the higher the solution magnitude impedance results. An experimental campaign, conducted on eggplants, is reported in order to illustrate the electrochemical characterization results.

4.1 Insulin Measurement in Diabetology

Diabetes is one of the most widely spread non-communicable chronic diseases worldwide. As amply treated in the first chapter, for diabetic patients, a full control of blood glucose level is a challenge with a relevant clinical, social, and economic impact.

The more and more promising technology advances in blood glucose self-monitoring provide new devices, which are smaller, faster, more reliable, and easier to use, as well as with reduced blood sample. However, the demand for non-invasive analytical methods increases more and more to achieve effective

DOI: 10.1201/9781003170143-4

glucose monitoring in diabetics. In particular, an accurate real-time glucose monitoring is required in combination with a long-term stability.

The Artificial Pancreas (AP, Fig. 4.1) represents a promising response to this demand; however, it presents more than a few limitations. The AP, known also as closed-loop control of Blood Glucose Concentration (BGC), mainly consists of a glucose sensor, control algorithms, and an insulin infusion device (Insulin Pump). The glucose sensor, generally placed on the arm, is fundamental in order to monitor the variability over time of BGC, to tailor insulin dosage, and to measure the efficacy of therapy after administration.

Continuous glucose monitoring is performed in the interstitial fluid, thus, it is associated with a time delay implicit from plasma concentration. Above all, the latency (on average 6.8 min and up to almost 10 min [164]) introduced by semi-non-invasive glucose meters, requires the AP external input to improve the glycaemia regulation. The AP loop is closed automatically in case of basal insulin administration; on the other hand, in case of bolus administration, the system cannot react instantaneously to the quick BGC variation caused by food ingestion. Thus, to maintain glycaemic levels in an acceptable range, external inputs are needed, such as: Total Daily Dose of insulin (TDD), carbintake, basal/bolus ratio, basal segments, carbohydrate-to-insulin ratio (CIR), target range, insulin sensitivity factor (ISF) and, insulin duration of action. Especially, the levels of ISF and insulin duration are fixed during the initial calibration of the device (AP or insulin pump), carried out usually more than once a day. However, these parameters may significantly change depending on the kinetics of the insulin absorption.

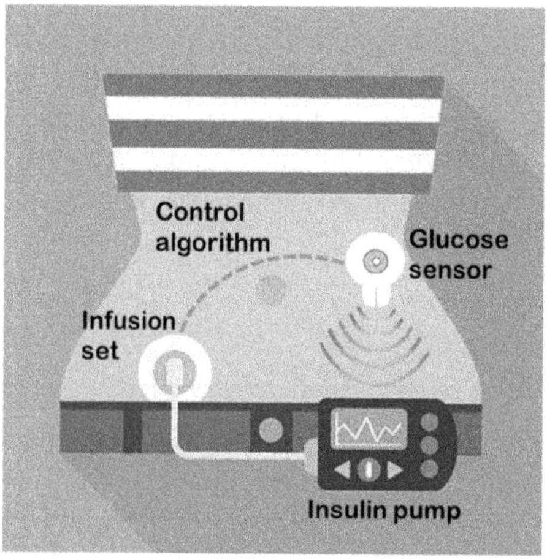

FIGURE 4.1
Schematic representation of AP.

Moreover, commercial insulin pumps assess the amount of glucose in the blood in order to identify the insulin absorption curve. In this manner, suitable software packages (e.g., Bolus Wizard [165]) determine the insulin to be administered during the day. Nevertheless, the amount of glucose in the blood is not a direct indication of the punctual insulin absorption.

This issue is particularly evident in case of skin alteration, such as lipo-hypertrophic nodules [166]. These nodules are associated with poor metabolic control and with a considerable intra-individual glycaemic instability (Fig. 4.2). Actually, different classes of drugs, used in insulin therapies, have a delayed and variable absorption if injected into lipohypertrophic nodules [6, 167].

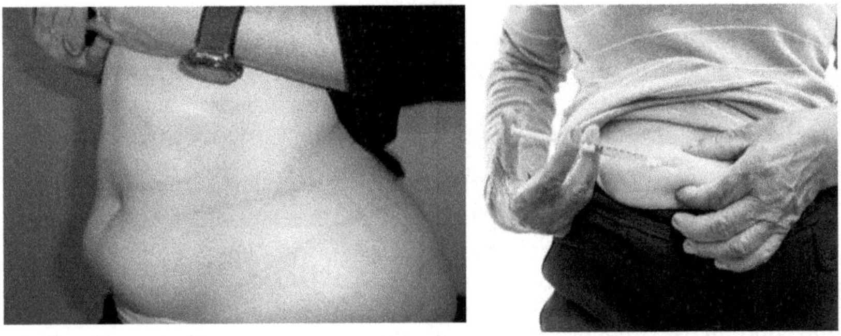

FIGURE 4.2
Two visible lipohypertrophic lesions below the navel on the left [6], and typical abdomen insulin injection on the right.

These problems affect also advanced automated diabetic therapy, where the identification of optimal doses and administration intervals are estimated on empirical basis. Thus, a proper insulin bolus administration is not ensured by a real-time monitoring of the insulin amount actually absorbed, namely bioavailable [168]. Unfortunately, to date, the main methods for assessing insulin bioavailability, i.e., the fraction (%) of administered drug that reaches the systemic circulation, are invasive or have high latency [169].

Therefore, a non-invasive method turns out to be extremely useful for monitoring the disappearance of insulin from the administration site. Furthermore, the possibility to estimate the insulin disappearance curve could provide a sound basis for the analysis of personalized therapies in different conditions of use, and could improve the effectiveness of the bolus wizard for diabetic patients as well.

4.2 Method

A measurement method for monitoring in real-time insulin bioavailability will be illustrated in the following subsections.

4.2.1 Basic Ideas

BIA might be considered as a potential method for monitoring the progressive disappearance of a drug, subcutaneously administered, in order to obtain an indicator for the individual absorption rate. According to the well-known concept of bioimpedance [170, 171], a tissue is considered as an electrolytic solution containing a certain number of cells. A solution is a homogeneous mixture of two or more substances. An electrolyte solution is a solution that generally contains ions, atoms or molecules, and it is electrically conductive. The substances that are dissolved are called solutes. The solute amount in a solution is evaluated by solution impedance measurement. In the same way, the insulin amount in the biological tissue is assessed by the caused impedance variation. On the basis of these principles, a measurement method for measuring insulin bioavailabilty exploits the following basic ideas [2]:

- The insulin bioavailability is a physical quantity that can be measured indirectly. Indeed, it is assessed starting from the administration volume of insulin disappearance in the biological tissue over time;
- BIA is a non-invasive measurement and the disappearance of a certain insulin amount (ml) generates an equivalent impedance change, measured in the administration volume. The impedance phase is not considered in the measurement due to its low linearity and monotonicity. Therefore, the result is expressed only by impedance magnitude;
- The relationship between impedance variation and insulin decrease can be properly modelled by a linear relationship [7, 172];
- A linear model for each subject is determined for every specific condition (personalized medicine) during each administration. Thus, both inter-individual and intra-individual reproducibility of the bioavailability measures is guaranteed and improved;
- The personalized linear model is characterized metrologically in order to assess the resolution, the reproducibility and the sensibility of the insulin amount evaluation;
- Electrochemical cell studies and an experimental campaign on eggplants were carried out in [7], by demonstrating the impedance magnitude variability as a function of the insulin amount variation (ml) in a solution.

The purpose of the measurement method presented below is to discriminate the electrical effects of active ingredient of the drug administered in the subcutaneous tissue, by testing drugs with different insulin concentration levels.

4.2.2 Measurement Method

The method for measuring the amount of insulin actually conveyed under the skin is illustrated in Fig. 4.3. It is based on the following main phases.

Firstly, the impedance measurement is measured by sending a sinusoidal current stimulus, with a specific amplitude and frequency, to the tissue under test, where the insulin in injected. Then, throughout the analog signal conditioning, the corresponding voltage drop, through the voltage meter, is assessed. The insulin is injected at known steps of known amount by an insulin pump or an insulin pen, used as reference for the calibration. Thus, the corresponding impedance variation, measured step by step, allows to perform a personalized model identification (insulin appearance model). During the insulin administration, the personalized individual model parameters are assessed during the off-line metrological characterization. Then a fault detection technique is applied to check if the personalized individual model parameters are within the uncertainty limits range. Thus, the insulin absorbed by the tissue is measured, through an assessment of the impedance variation according to an insulin disappearance model (bioavailability monitoring).

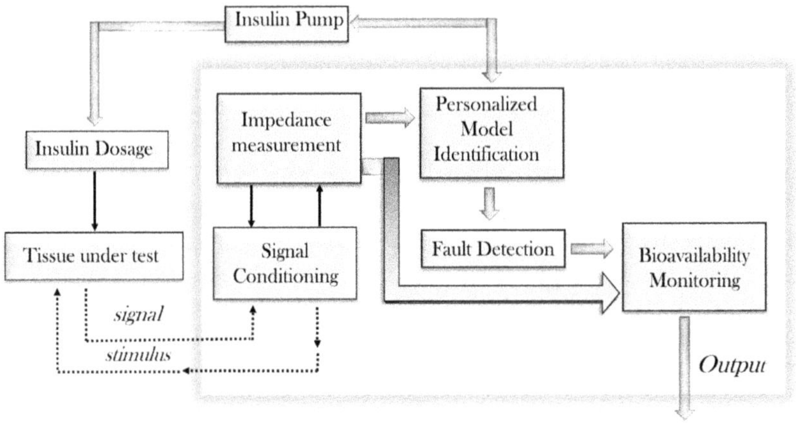

FIGURE 4.3
Insulin measurement method phases.

4.2.3 Setup

The instrument used in this application is the Drug Under Skin Meter (DUSM) already presented in the previous chapter. The DUSM is essentially an impedance spectroscope flexible for several utilizations, including clinical application.

The new application of DUSM in this section aims to analyze the tissue impedance evolution over time, which is associated to the progressive decrease of insulin concentration in subcutaneous tissue. This trend is highly related to drug impedance. The main purpose, which is quite different from the previous study, is to measure the variation of only one ingredient of the employed solution, but a sensitivity problem arises. In order to check if the instrument sensitive is appropriate, the operations are carried out in a controlled environment under favourable conditions, that is, using an electrochemical cell.

To this aim, the DUSM is equipped with a sensor based on 2-pole electrochemical cell technology. The electrochemical cell requires two electrodes of the same metal, which build up an electric circuit of two double-layers in parallel, surrounded by an electrolyte solution which fills the gap. Electrochemical cells convert chemical energy into electricity, so the sensor can realize cell analysis and evaluation through measurement of electrochemical signals. With the aim of converting the conductance readings into conductivity results, the related measuring chain needs to be calibrated. The value of cell constant is assessed under specific operating conditions, since the determination of conductivity is possible once the cell constant is known. The cell constant can be experimentally determined using reference solutions with exactly known conductivity. The cell constant is a multiplier constant specific to a conductivity sensor; it is directly proportional to the distance separating the two conductive plates and, inversely proportional to their surface area. The measured current is multiplied by the cell constant to determine the electrical conductivity of the solution.

To assess the cell constant, an experiment using a standard solution of known conductivity referenced to temperature, Hanna HI7031L, was used. It was subject to measure at a temperature of 26.2 °C, with stimulus signal amplitude of 520 mV and frequency of 1 kHz. The resulting cell constant was 0.742. Conductivity is measured by determining the amount of current that flows between two electrodes when the volume of the solution is known. The electrical conductivity of a solution, represents the charge transport capacity of the ions and it depends also on external factors such as temperature or pressure.

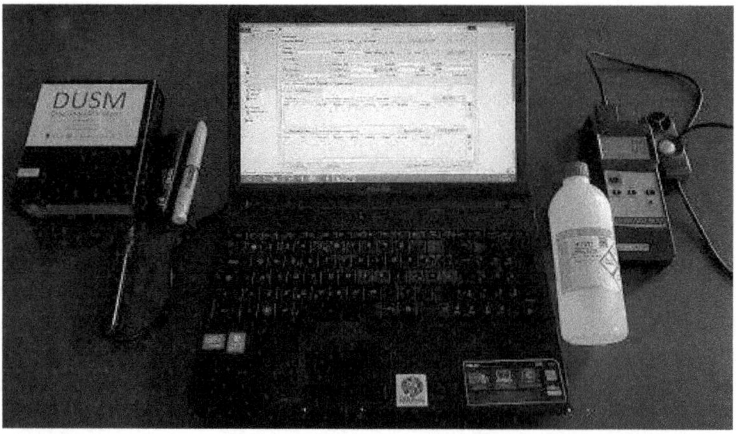

FIGURE 4.4
The DUSM in electrochemical cell configuration [7].

4.2.4 Insulin Solution Electrical Characterization

To handle the blood glucose concentration, insulin injection is the principal treatment of adults and children with diabetes mellitus, who require insulin for the maintenance of normal glucose homeostasis. Several different kinds of insulin, with various pharmacokinetic properties, are available on the market. The dose and the type of insulin should be determined carefully by the physician, according to the requirement of the patient.

The insulin electrical behaviour can be revealed by impedance measurements; this latter were carried out on twenty-two distinct insulin solutions, realized using two different pharmaceutical preparations as solute and a saline solvent. The pharmaceutical products, chosen for the experiments, presented opposite pharmacokinetics proprieties. On one hand, there was the Abasaglar insulin by Lilly, a basal insulin which contains insulin glargine, an insulin analogue with a prolonged duration of action. It is administered subcutaneously and provide a smooth, peakless, and predictable concentration/time profile, with a prolonged duration of action. The longer duration of action of subcutaneous insulin glargine is directly related to its slower rate of absorption and supports once daily administration. On the other hand, there was the Humalog insulin by Lilly; namely rapid-acting insulin, it contains Lispro insulin, with a rapid onset of action (approximately 15 minutes). It also has a shorter duration of activity (2 to 5 hours) when given subcutaneously. The pharmacokinetics of Lispro reflects a compound that is rapidly absorbed.

For each pharmaceutical preparation, eleven solutions were arranged, with concentration levels in saline solvent varying from 0.00 to 100.00 U/ml with 10.00 U/ml steps. In particular, each ml contains 100 units of Lispro insulin that is equivalent to 3.50 mg, meanwhile for insulin glargine each ml contains 100 units, equivalent to 3.64 mg. The room temperature was of 20.0 °C, the stimulus signal presents the same set for calibration. For each data set, the best fitting curve equation is reported in Fig. 4.5.

The results highlight, in both the cases, a direct relationship between insulin concentration and impedance magnitude, well modelled by a 4th degree polynomial. The higher the concentration level of insulin is the higher the solution magnitude impedance results.

4.3 Method Feasibility

In this section, the DUSM effectiveness, experimentally proven, is illustrated for assessing the insulin concentration within a subcutaneous tissue. Also in this case, eggplants were used to emulate electrical human tissue behaviour.

The mere replication of the experiment realized in the electrochemical cell did not was possible. Differently from an electrochemical cell, a biological

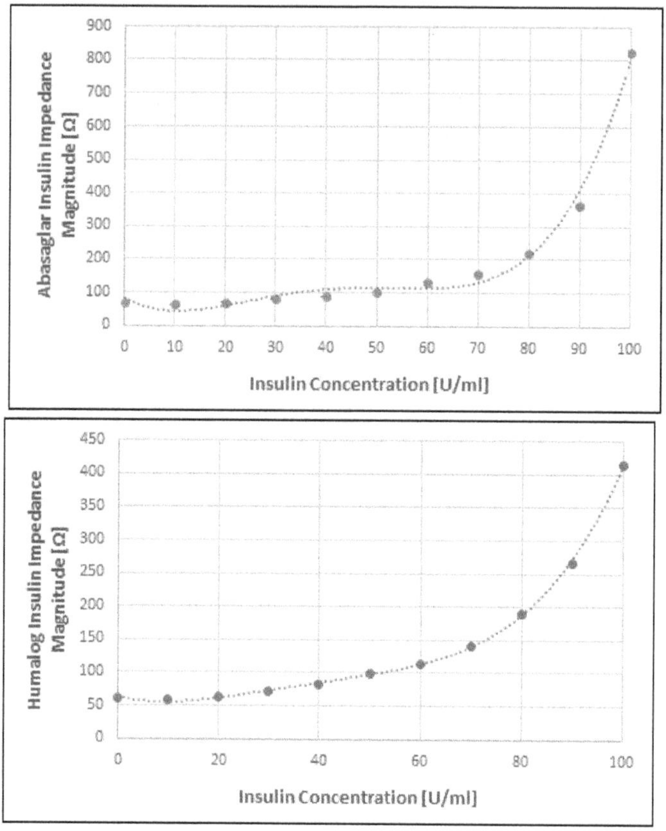

FIGURE 4.5
Measured impedance magnitude at varying concentration for insulin solution of Abasaglar (up) and Humalog (down) and fitting curves equations [7].

tissue does not represent a neutral and controlled environment. In fact, it cannot be emptied of the previously injected solution to introduce a different concentration. Nor can it be reproduced in replicas capable of only introducing a systematic perturbation to the measurement. The biological tissue, rather, is the source of inter-subjective non-reproducibility, which overcomes the impact of the changing insulin concentration. Therefore, the experiment is to be adapted as explained below.

Six constant volumes of a solution with two different insulin concentrations were injected in the same eggplant. Considering the linear dependence of the impedance variation with respect to the increment of drug amount [2], the effect of insulin concentration on the magnitude of the linearity coefficient was assessed. The composition of the solution, as well as the distance between the two electrodes and their size, were selected according to the following

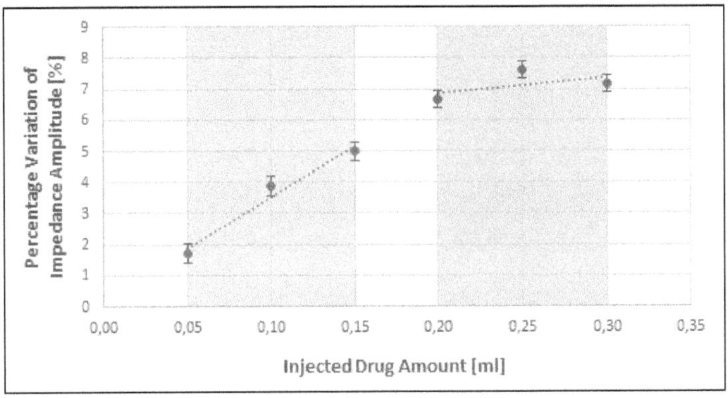

FIGURE 4.6
Impedance magnitude percentage variation at varying injected volume for two different insulin concentration solutions: 10.00 U/ml (blue) and 100.00 U/ml (red) [7].

considerations. In particular, two surface cutaneous electrodes, with total area of 3.64 cm^2 with an inter-electrodes gap of 1.4 cm, deliver a sinusoidal current. The selected signal, generated by the impedance spectroscope, presented 100 mV amplitude and 1 kH frequency, respectively. The initial three injections were realised with Humalog insulin solution at a concentration of 10.00 U/ml (Fig. 4.6, in blue), by three steps of 0.05 ml. The other three injections were realised with the same solution volumes at concentration of 100.00 U/ml (Fig. 4.6, in red). The impedance values of the two solutions are significantly different, and this determined two distinct decreasing ratesof impedance magnitude of the tissue. For all the 10 samples, the six points of impedance magnitude percentage variation are separately fitted in groups of three, and two lines with different average slope are obtained. The slope of lines best fitting the second group is, on average, 3.53 times lower than those of the lines best fitting the first ones. The results concerning the slope variation are compatible with the measurements obtained by the electrochemical cell.

4.3.1 Discussion

In this chapter, a measurement method, tested at University of Naples Federico II, is proved to be able to discriminate two equal drug volumes with different insulin concentration, at a known depth, in an eggplant. The volumes and concentration are typical of diabetes treatments. In the next chapters, further in-vivo experiments will highlight that the device can precisely discriminate between volume with different insulin concentrations injected in the subcutaneous tissue, with a suitable resolution (defined by standard insulin treatments) and excluding intra-subjective variability affection.

5

Insulin Meter

CONTENTS

An insulin meter, based on an on-chip transducer, for real-time non-invasive monitoring of insulin absorption is presented in this chapter. The instrument, prototyped by using all off-the-shelf components, analyzes the electrical bioimpedance in the frequency domain and its variations over time. Once insulin has been injected in the tissue under test by the insulin pump in known doses, the transducer measures step by step the corresponding impedance variation. Thus, the insulin meter carries out a personalized model identification. The personalized model of insulin appearance is specific for each subject. It is identified and validated during each insulin administration. Thus, inter-and-intra individual reproducibility is enhanced. Then, the insulin bioavailability over time is assessed indirectly by monitoring its time-dependent disappearance from the administration volume of biological tissue. The concept, the whole system design, along with the hardware and software realization are described hereafter. Finally, the instrument calibration is reported.

5.1 Design

Starting from the feasibility shown in the previous chapter, the design of an instrument for measuring insulin absorption is presented below. In the previous chapters, an instrument able to assess the amount of drug transdermal delivered into the tissue, namely the DUSM, was presented. This time, instead of assessing the appearance of the drug, the *Insulin Meter* is able to

DOI: 10.1201/9781003170143-5

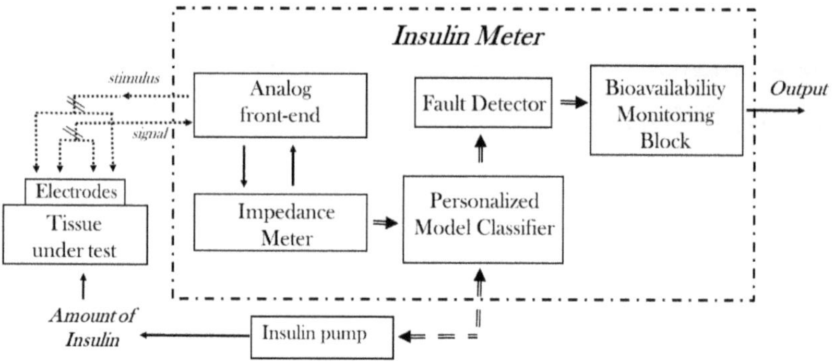

FIGURE 5.1
Architecture of the Insulin Meter [8].

measure the disappearance of the drug from the injection site. Thus, the drug bioavailability is assessed indirectly.

5.1.1 Architecture

The architecture of the Insulin Meter is highlighted in Fig. 5.1. Four pre-gelled *Electrodes*, two amperometric and two voltmetric, are applied on a specific body area, the *Tissue Under Test*, where the insulin is administrated. A given sinusoidal current is imposed, and a corresponding voltage drop is measured by the *Impedance Meter* through the *Analog front-end.*

When the *Insulin Pump* administers the insulin amount at fixed steps, the transducer measures the corresponding impedance variation. Subsequently, starting from these measurements, the Insulin Meter identifies a personalized model experimentally through the *Personalized Model Classifier.*

The parameters of the identified model are checked by the *Fault Detector* to verify if they fall within the uncertainty limits fixed during the off-line metrological characterization. If so, the *Bioavalaibility Monitoring block* assesses the insulin amount systemically absorbed (and, therefore, disappeared from the tissue under test), by measuring the impedance variation.

5.1.2 Operation

The Insulin Meter operates according to the following steps:

- *Electrodes Application*: the four-electrodes configuration is used to soften the impact of the electrolytic gel on the impedance drift. Adhesive pre-gelled electrodes FIAB PG500 (Vicchio, Florence, Italy) [149] are employed to reduce the movement artifacts and to improve the the electrodes-skin contact. Moreover, a personalized 3-D printed support in Thermoplastic polyurethane (TPU) is used to stabilize the measurement setup and to improve the placement on the anatomical site;

- *Reproducibility Enhancement*: the average of the impedance magnitude acquired at each measure cycle is used to reduce the single measurement uncertainty. As concern the inter-individual reproducibility, each individual exhibits a different behaviour of the tissue impedance, due especially to the variability of the stratum corneum thickness and hydration. The reproducibility is improved by normalizing the impedance average to its pre-administration value;
- *Model Construction*: the impedance is measured at the frequency of 1 kHz after each step of insulin administration. The calibration model is determined from the injection process and it associates the impedance variation to the insulin amount. The relationship between the impedance variation and the drug amount is well modelled by a linear relationship (Fig. 5.2). During the injection phase, this model is identified both for each subject and for each particular physiological condition of the same subject. Therefore, the intra-subjective and inter-subjective reproducibility is improved;
- *Fault Detection*: a compatibility check is implemented between the linear model identified and the tolerance range resulted from the initial metrological characterization of the insulinometer;
- *Bioavailability Monitoring*: the impedance variations are measured over time to assess the corresponding insulin absorption (insulin disappearance) through the linear model built in the injection phase (insulin appearance). In the following subsection, a specific focus on bioavailability measurement is presented.

5.1.3 Bioavailability Monitoring

Increasing gradually the amount of drug while measuring impedance variations allows to identifying a custom relationship for the specific tissue under test. An example of a typical model built after the insulin injection is presented in Fig. 5.2. In the same figure, the relationship between the amount of drug, injected by the insulin pump in known steps, and the percentage impedance variation is highlighted by the linear regression line. This model represents the insulin appearance model. It can be employed for monitoring the insulin disappearance, due to the absorption by human body, and thus the bioavailability. The model, specific for the subject and the distinct injection site, allows to improve significantly inter- and intra-individual reproducibility.

The insulin appearance model is built during the injection for assessing the amount of the absorbed drug. After the insulin injection, at the instant t_0, an impedance measurement detects a percentage variation of -12 % compared to the impedance value before injection (pink dot in the top of Fig. 5.3). The

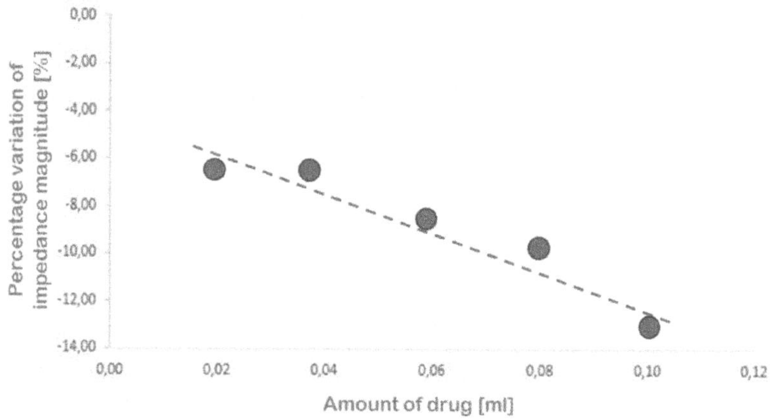

FIGURE 5.2
Insulin appearance model building: linear relationship between the amount of insulin and the percentage impedance variation.

appearance model allows to estimate around 0.09 ml of drug still in situ, and, therefore, not absorbed (yellow dot). An inverse model of insulin appearance is used in the absorption (disappearance) phase. At the instant t_1 (bottom of Fig. 5.3), an impedance measurement detects a percentage variation of -6 % compared to the impedance value before injection. In this case, 0.02 ml of drug are estimated to be still in situ. Consequently, almost all the insulin was absorbed.

5.2 Realization

This section presents the design and the characterization of the Insulin Meter, prototyped by using all off-the-shelf components. The instrument is able to analyze the electrical bioimpedance in the frequency domain and its variations over time. The system design as a whole, employing a tetra-polar electrode configuration, includes a motherboard EVALADUCM350-REV A, and a daughterboard BIO3Z Vers.A, both components of Analog Device [173].

5.2.1 Hardware, Firmware, and Software

Part of the equipment employed in the Insulin Meter has already been used in different configurations and experimental tests by the Authors, as described in the previous chapters.

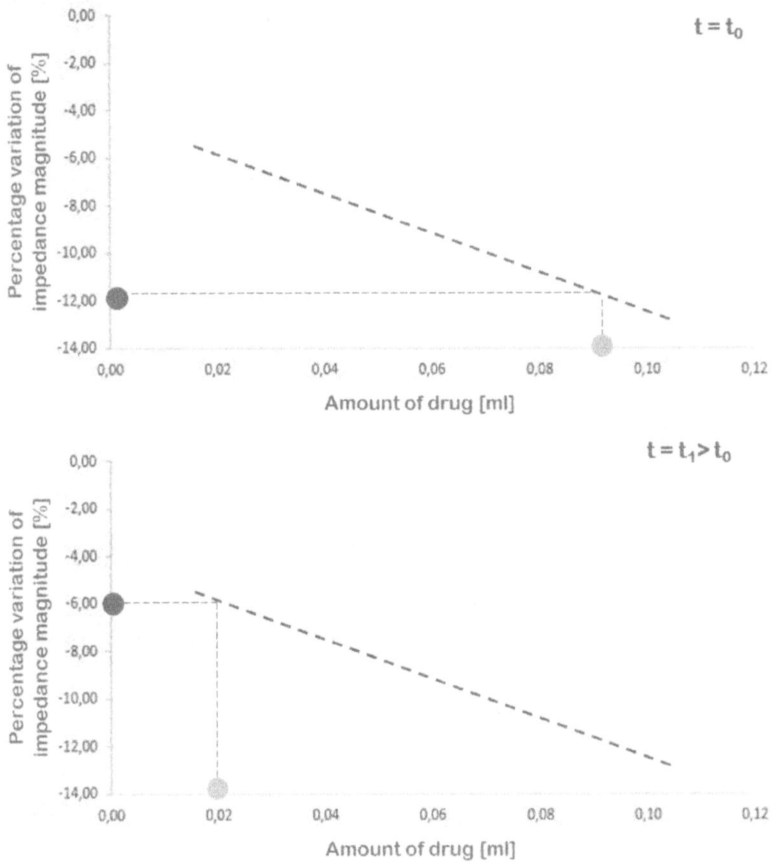

FIGURE 5.3
Personalized model of insulin appearance used to evaluate the disappearance of insulin.

Hardware The instrument version, here presented, consists of a black rigid outer case, specifically designed and 3D-printed in order to guarantee the insulation of all the components. The case contains a motherboard, the Eval-AduCM350 EBZ Vers.A, equipped with an analog front-end and a processor ARM Cortex-M3 at 16 MHz, specifically designed for high-precision data acquisition. The motherboard imposes the sinusoidal input signal with its 16-bit DAC, and it is able to convert the sensed current signal into a voltage signal by means of its 16-bit to 160 kSa/s ADC. The motherboard performs a Discrete Fourier Transform (DFT) on 2048 points, which is used for ac impedance measurements. It presents the real and imaginary parts of a complex result [170, 171].

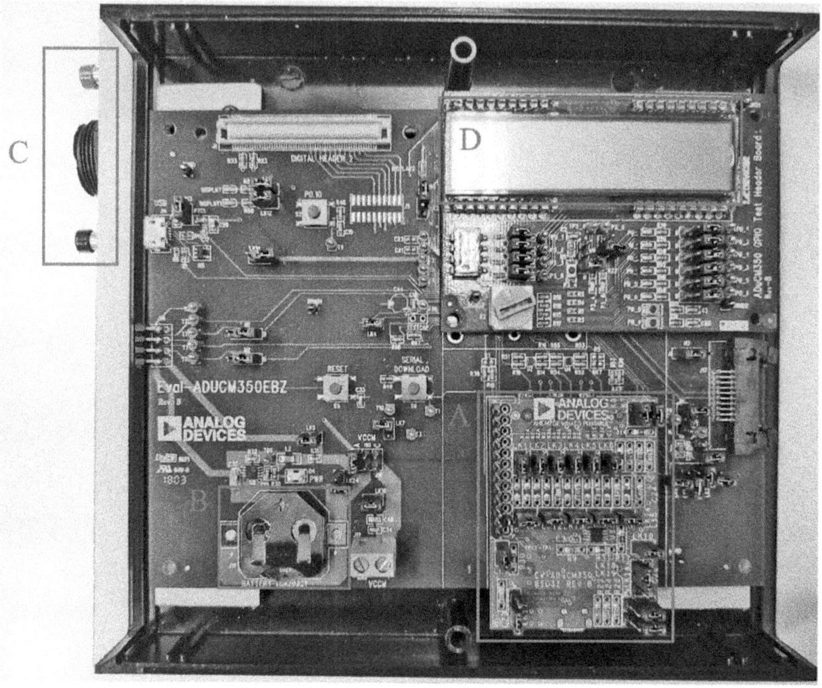

FIGURE 5.4
Prototype board of the insulin meter: motherboard ADuCM350 Vers.A with (A) daughterboard BIO3Z for 4-wire bioimpedance measurement, (B) battery, (C) ON and Reset buttons, and (D) display [8].

The motherboard (Fig. 5.4) presents a slot for the daughterboard of signal conditioning. The daughterboard "4-Wire Bio Impedance Configuration 4W-BIO3Z" of Fig. 5.4 (A) can performs 4-wire measurements. The Insulin Meter provides a collection of power modes and features. The three main supply options include: USB cable, battery, and 3.3 V via external transformer and wall socket. The battery solution, shown in Fig. 5.4 (B), might be adopted when the device is used as an actual portable system, potentially applicable in several e-health scenarios, and for home-care of chronic patients, as well as for continuous daily monitoring (i.e., holter monitoring). At this aim, the user can verify, at any time, the measurement process by means of an 8-digit ADuCM350-GPIO-REV-B LCD of the Analog Device, shown in Fig. 5.4 (D), and a selector.

Finally, the board is connected to the biological tissue under test through four electrodes. One of the key challenges in bioimpedance measurement systems is the electrode placement. The design of a bioimpedance device cannot avoid to consider and reduce the adverse effects connected to electrode polarization, the high contact impedance, the noise of the interface, and the artefacts due to movements along with contact problems. The electrodes represent the electrochemical interface needed to connect the biological medium with the measuring equipment, both for the voltage detection and the injection of current. For bioimpedance measurements on the human body, described in this book, the electrodes FIAB PG500 are used, where the electrode-skin contact consists of a metal flexible electrode, and adhesive and conductive solid gel Ag-AgCl electrode, with an electrolyte based on Cl^-.

In this case, a quadruple electrodes configuration is adopted, where two stimulation electrodes inject the current, while two detection electrodes acquire the associated voltage drop produced by the current circulation. When the biological medium is the human body, strict international safety standards must be respected in order to avoid any possible hazard or harmful effect. In particular, the standard IEC 60601-1 [147] for the safety of electromedical equipment with the patient's active part indicates the limits of leakage currents under normal and faulty conditions. The injected current must be monitored to avoid exceeding the established limits, which are divided into two main ranges, depending on whether the stimulus frequency f_e is lower or higher than 1 kHz. When the frequency is lower that 1 kHz, the maximum RMS current allowed by the standard is 10 μA.

$$f <= 1\ kHz, \qquad I_{MAX} = 10\ \mu A$$

$$f > 1\ kHz, \qquad I_{MAX} = \frac{f_e}{1000Hz} * 10\ \mu A$$

The insulin meter remains always below the thresholds imposed by the standard due to an additional suitable resistors and capacitors located on the doughterboard in series with the unknown impedance, as shown in Fig. 5.5 in red. Indeed, the series of three resistors, of 3 kΩ equivalent value, keeps the current peak below 8 μA.

Firmware and software Despite the Analog Device provides libraries for basic operation exploiting the BIO3Z board, such as 4-wires impedance measurements, a new firmware is to be developed for the transducer. A set of ten different programs is created to make the measurement faster and more user-friendly. The analog front-end is initialized only at the measurement start, allowing so to increase the throughput. Whereas, the data transmission is postponed at the measurement, because all the data are saved in the internal flash memory. In doing so, the acquisition time is reduced down to 34 %. Up to 7500 16-bytes measurements can be saved on the transducer memory spaces of 120 kB. The collected data can be downloaded by connecting the instrument to the PC via the COM port with the UART management protocol. During the debug, to start or stop a measurement by hand, two easily-accessible ON and Reset buttons are available. Meanwhile, the display allows the user to view the current program and the current measurement number program (Fig. 5.4 D).

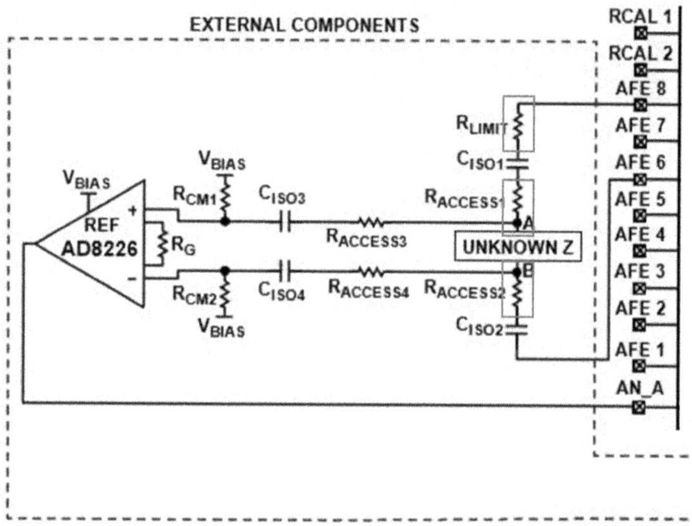

FIGURE 5.5
Daughterboard schematic with the three resistors in series to limit the current (RCALi, input for the calibration resistor, AN_A, the auxiliary channels, and AFEi, inputs for the analog front-end) [5].

When the Insulin Meter is connected to the PC via the COM port, a user-friendly interface is available. The Insulin Meter is configured by means of the user interface illustrated in Fig. 5.6, developed by using different user controls (label, textbox, lists, combo box, etc.). The user can define the information on the measurement session to be performed. In particular, the user can collect the personal data of the patients enrolled in the study, such as age, sex, ethnicity, skin fototype, as well as environment and experimental settings (e.g., room temperature and humidity, the used drug, and the injection site). The interface allows to set the working frequency and amplitude and the number of measurements. Moreover, the data received by the device are properly processed and displayed. Finally, the database of collected data is available for further processing, research, visualization, and plotting.

5.3 Calibration

The Insulin Meter was characterized metrologically, firstly, (i) in laboratory, by means of a direct comparison against reference impedance; then, (ii) in-vitro, on eggplants, (iii) ex-vivo, on pigs, and, finally, (iv) preliminarily in-vivo,

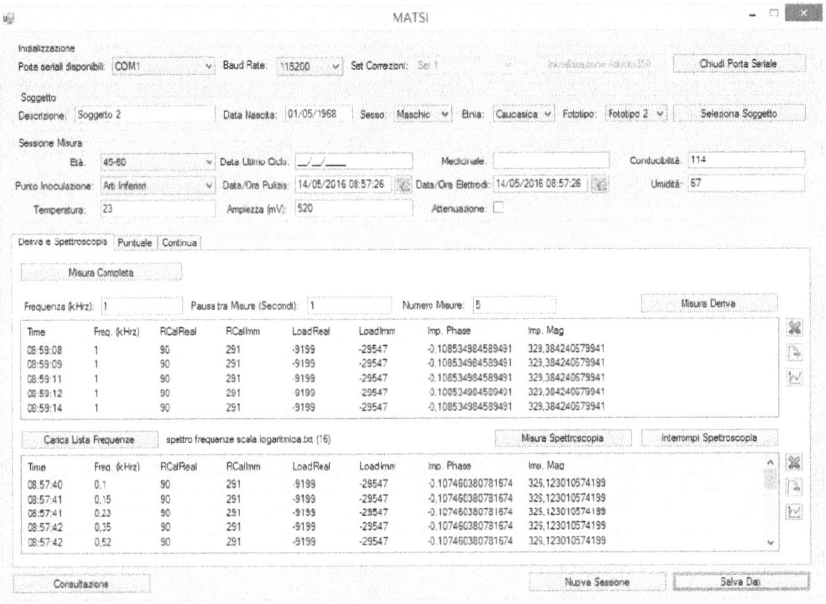

FIGURE 5.6
User Interface of the Insulin Meter [9].

on a human subject, through insulin infiltration. This chapter intends to focus attention on the laboratory characterization, while the following chapters will deal deeply with the other tests.

Experimental setup

In laboratory test, the Insulin Meter was compared directly with a more accurate instrument, the Agilent 4263B LCR Meter, used as reference. This latter is specifically designed for both component evaluation and fundamental impedance testing. Meanwhile, a Decade Resistor 1433-M and a Standard Capacitor Type 509-Fm, both of General Radio, realized an equivalent parallel circuit between a capacitor [0.5 nF] and a variable resistor (42 to 2500) Ω.

Calibration

The measurements were carried out in chambers where environment factors were controlled; in particular, the temperature was 23 °C and the relative humidity 50 %. The impedance magnitude was measured for a set of frequency points chosen in the 100 Hz to 20 kHz frequency range. In particular, 32 measurements were carried out, for each resistor value, at the frequency of 100 Hz, 120 Hz, 10000 Hz, 20000 Hz, by generating for each point a sinusoidal waveform of amplitude 100 mV. The mean and the standard deviation of the impedance magnitude of the of the RC loop were assessed, at each selected resistor value. The resistor value varied in a linear sequential manner within (42 to 2500) Ω.

Results

Considering the nominal values calculated for the RC loop at 1 kHz, both the instruments, the Agilent 4263B LCR Meter and the Insulin Meter, present an impedance variation trend compatible with the nominal one. Fig. 5.7 shows the impedance variation measured at 1 kHz by the instruments, at varying the resistor value of the RC loop.

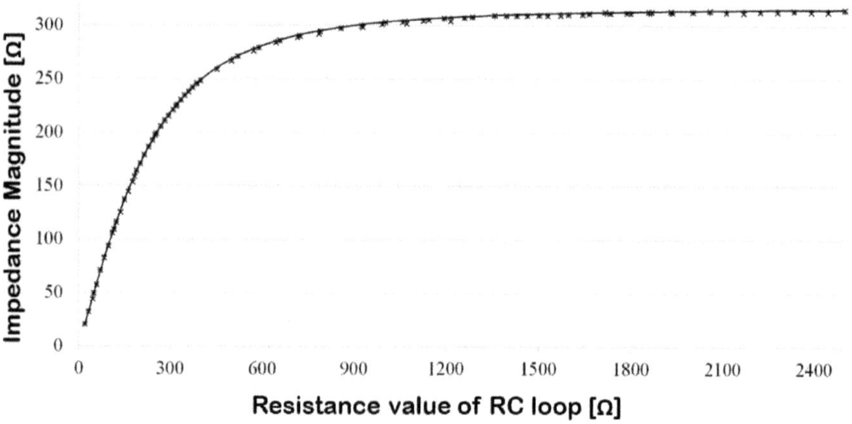

FIGURE 5.7
Impedance magnitude at 1 kHz at varying the resistance value of the RC loop: theoretical trend (continuous line), insulin meter (×), and reference LCR Meter (+) [8].

6

Measurement Method for Orthopaedics

CONTENTS

This chapter presents the most important tasks to be faced in orthopaedic measurements for realizing the personalized model of parts of the human body, with a specific reference to the knee, one of the most complex joints of the body. A subject-specific Finite Element Method (FEM) model allows to optimize the electrodes design and adhesion, leading to a better understanding of the human body behaviour. Thus, this permits to evaluate the injuries extent as well as the therapy progress. Indeed, the personalized model will be used to enhance the inter-individual reproducibility of a measurement method for monitoring Non-Steroidal Anti-Inflammatory Drugs (NSAIDs) after transdermal delivery in the clinical practice. In particular, the following sections present the anatomical structure of the knee joint and its dielectric proprieties, provided by the Cole-Cole expression. Furthermore, on this basis, the numerical model of the human knee is illustrated. The model is based on the Finite Element Analysis of a set of Partial Differential Equations derived by the Direct Current formulation of Maxwell equation in the frequency domain. The model effectiveness is increased also by considering the presence of lossy dielectric materials characterized by relaxation phenomena.

6.1 Measurement Concepts for Orthopaedics

One of the main consequences of external trauma are direct injuries: simple contusion, or even muscle failure, or bone fractures, according to trauma force and the muscles state of contraction. By and large, bone fractures can occur

DOI: 10.1201/9781003170143-6

under traumatic events or even non-traumatic condition, due to pathological status as osteoporosis, arthritis, bone cancer, and so on.

One of the most critical components of the human body, important for carrying out daily activity, is the knee joint. Unfortunately, the knee joint is often subject to injuries (bone injuries, sprains, ligaments strain, and tendinitis) or to degenerative disease, like osteoarthritis, rheumatoid arthritis, and other inflammatory disorders leading to chronic pain.

The therapy suggested for several of these pathologies often includes topical administration of a NonSteroidal Anti-Inflammatory Drugs (NSAIDs). These medicines are widely used to relieve pain, reduce inflammation, and bring down to a normal temperature. According to the American Academy of Orthopaedic Surgeons (JAAOS), [174], NSAIDs are ranked as the most efficient nonsurgical osteoarthritis knee treatment, low-cost and nearly safe, for enhancing functionality and providing pain relief. They are a broad group of drugs from a number of different classes. They are effective analgesics, commonly available as tablets, capsules, suppositories, creams, gels and injection, although their chemical structures are different. For the treatment of acute pain and local muscle inflammation, they are commonly administered by transdermal drug delivery. Topically they are applied to intact skin in painful area in the form of a gel, cream, spray or patch. They penetrate the skin, pervade tissues or joints in depth, and reduce the inflammation process [175,176].

Simply put, a generic drug can be defined as a chemical substance of known structure, other than nutrient included in ordinary diet, which once administrated to a living organism, causes a change in an organism's physiology. When a pharmaceutical drug is administrated to treat, cure, prevent or ameliorate any symptoms of a disease, or in general to promote people's health, it is best known as medication or medicine. The final medical drug is a combination of different chemical substances defined by a pharmaceutical formulation. According to the IUPAC definition, pharmacokinetics is the "process of the uptake of drugs by the body, the biotransformation they undergo, the distribution of the drugs and their metabolites in the tissues, and the elimination of the drugs and their metabolites from the body over a period of time". It is beyond doubt that, despite of the promising advances in the biomedical engineering field, there is an increasing demand for real-time non-invasive monitoring solutions of drug pharmacokinetics . Hence, bioimpedance measurement represents a valid answer to this request. In particular, BIA can be employed in pharmacological investigation and pharmacokinetics studies [141]. It might be considered as a potential method to monitor the progressive disappearance of a drug, subcutaneously administered, in order to obtain an indicator for the individual absorption rate. So, by exploring subcutaneous tissue in a non-invasive way, personalized therapies are obtained. For transdermal delivery, standardized methods for measuring the drug actually penetrated during the treatment are missing. Especially for orthopaedic treatments, where drugs as NSAIDs actually absorbed and the related efficacy of the treatment are empirically assessed according to the operator experience.

Nowadays, the dynamic of drug applied and targeted in local skin sites is less clear and studied, compared to the systemic acting drugs. In fact, the main focus is on the evaluation of the drug amount that reaches the general circulation for systemically acting drugs given by, for example, the oral or invasive administration. In particular, there are still problems in correlating the availability of a topically applied drug in the skin, and its therapeutic activity at the site of action, to the absorption rate.

The concentration of drug which diffuses into the underlying tissue can be assessed by several invasive approaches, such as: blood analysis, plasma concentration, and skin biopsy. The biopsy is accurate and reliable, but, on the other hand, it is an extremely invasive approach and so unacceptable for routine use. Instead, a non-invasive solution like BIA would be applied in everyday clinical practice.

Overall, it is difficult to quantify the amount of drug within the skin for topical products, also owing to the intra-individual (different body areas, skin conditions, psychological conditions, and so on), as well as to inter-individual factors (sex, age, ethnicity, and so on) [177]. Moreover, the absorption kinetics, the efficacy, and the bioavailability of topical drug are poorly understood, also due to pharmacokinetic measurements in blood, plasma, or urine, which are usually not appropriate because of the very-low concentrations achieved in these typical sampling compartments.

A characterization of the absorption process is crucial to both the design of improved drug delivery systems, and the definition of the pharmacokinetic as well as pharmacodynamics features, required for adjusting the dose progressively in pharmacology therapies [178]. In 2015, the European Medicine Agency already highlighted the critical demand to establish and define new methods for measuring the in-vivo administered of multiple classes of drugs.

At the present time, for in-vivo measurements and topical drug application, critical issues are linked to drug bioavailability and bioequivalence, which must be assessed typically via costly and time-consuming clinical studies [179]. In fact, in the case of topical medications, the equivalence between drugs is essentially based on the correlation of the active ingredient, by neglecting the importance of the excipients. In addition, there are no acceptable standard methods for the in-vivo assessment of local cutaneous bioavailability in humans after topical drug application [142, 180]. The systemic availability may not represent local cutaneous bioavailability accurately, as for transdermal or oral products, which are designed on the other hand, to deliver drug into the systemic circulation. The bioavailability is typically defined as the rate and amount of drug that reaches the general circulation from an administered dosage form. Thus, bioavailability assessment of a topical drug is crucial for both the transdermal delivery of pharmacological active drugs and a toxicological point of view.

Moreover, the evaluation of therapy effectiveness and recovery is provided by the physical examination of physicians, or using expensive, time-consuming, and harmful diagnostic imaging. Nowadays, the oldest but the most common technique used to diagnose fractured bones, joint dislocations, injuries and joint abnormalities is X-ray Radiography. This exam requires little time and no special preparation, but bulky and expensive equipment.

Therefore, a BIA system might represent a portable and effective device for quantifying joints health following an acute injury, both inside and outside the hospital, and a valuable help in rehabilitation process and monitoring. Besides that, BIA may provide information on the skin's reservoir function, essential to determinate the duration of the topical drug action [120], thus allowing to customize the therapy.

The purpose of the study presented below is to measure the amount of drug transported transdermally, for a local action, by minimizing systemic effects. The employed device measures this impedance, and consequently the amount of substance present in the subcutaneous tissue. The measurement relies on the introduction of a reference amount of conductive drug into a specific volume of biological tissue determining a variation in the equivalent bioimpedance [181].

Moreover, the assessment of drug transdermal delivered can enhance the performance of several drug vehiculation techniques. For example, an extensively used approach to improve transdermal drug delivery is iontophoresis, a type of electrotherapy, noninvasive, safe, and high-efficiency method of systemic and local drug delivery exploiting an electric field [182]. It turns out to be a technique fundamental for the treatment of osteoarticular pain, for reducing inflammation, knee pain, sciatica and arthrosis, as well as muscle strains. However, the exact time needed for the treatment and the amount of drug actually penetrated cannot be estimated. Hence, BIA can improve this treatment and really personalize the therapies. For all these reasons, regulatory agencies as well as physicians are seeking alternative methodologies to assess non-invasively the amount of topical drug. In particular, this is important for bioequivalence studies needed to relieve the burden for pursuing to commercialize useful products at competitive prices, and to reduce the time, the cost of treatments, but preserving the performance.

6.2 Knee Structure

The human knee is the component bearing the largest weight, and it is located between the two longest lever arms of body. Hence, it is the most stressed joint, and one of the most commonly injured. The joint pressure and dynamic loading vary during daily living activities; indeed, bones and muscles in healthy subjects adapt to their mechanical environment. Therefore, a healthy knee is valuable to properly fulfil daily functions and it significantly affects our quality of life.

Knee pain is a particularly widespread symptom; only in the United States, it interests nearly 40 million people reporting knee pain. It affects people of every age and sex, and its incidence increases considerably with ageing. Among young people, the most common causes of knee pain are acute and, in general, linked to accidental trauma, such as bruises and sprains, ligaments strain, and tendinitis. On the other hand, among older people, degenerative joint disease like osteoarthritis, rheumatoid arthritis, and other inflammatory disorders are the main causes of physical problems. However, the increase of pain severity dramatically decreases the quality of life and it might also lead to disability [183].

The human knee is one of the most complex joints of the human body, since its geometrical and anatomical structure allows the transmission of forces efficiently, and to bear the body weight and high stress. It has crucial biomechanical roles in gait, flexion, and extension of lower limbs.

The knee joint is a hinge type joint placed between femur, tibia, and patella. The femur is the longest bone of human body and represents the proximal part of the limb, or thigh. The head of the femur is a hemispherical surface that fits into the acetabulum of the hip joint, while the distal part of femur has two articular surfaces, named condyles, which are connected on the anterior side to patella through the patellar surface. The two femur condyles, meet the menisci placed over the tibial plateau (Fig. 6.1). Menisci are thickened disks shaped pad placed at the centre of the knee join. They protect the ends of the bones from rubbing on each other, and they also play a crucial role in shock absorption. The tibial plateau is located in the proximal part of the tibia, the long anterior leg bone, which together with fibula, positioned on the lateral side of the tibia, represent the bone structure of the lower part of the leg between the knee and the ankle [184].

By employing magnetic resonance imaging of 118 subjects, in [12], the tibia and femur dimensions were assessed; in particular, the average width of different plateau sections and the medial width and length of condyle are illustrated in Tab. 6.1 and in Fig. 6.1.

The patella is a flat bone that covers and shields the anterior articular surface of the knee joint, besides the tendon of the quadriceps femoris muscle attaches to the base of the patella.

The quadriceps is a large muscle group that collectively is one of the most powerful muscles in the body. It is located in the anterior compartment of the thigh and it represents the main bulk of the thigh. The other main muscles, illustrated in Fig. 6.2, are: (*i*) the gastrocnemius, the most superficial of the muscles in the posterior compartment which covers the entire posterior leg compartment; and (*ii*) the soleus, a large flat muscle which is the deepest lying of the superficial muscles, running from just below the knee to the heel and laying immediately deep to the gastrocnemius. It is worth highlighting that muscles thickness strongly relies on the subject sex and muscular tone. The same applies to bones, in fact the average values of bone dimensions in

TABLE 6.1
Typical values of tibia and femur dimensions for male and female. Tibial Plateau Width (TPW), tibial lateau Medial Length (ML), tibial plateau Medial Width (MW), Femur Condyle Width (FCW), medial Femoral condyle Length (FL), and Medial Femur Width (FW) [12].

	Bones (mm)	General	Male	Female
Tibia	TPW	74.9 ± 6.5	80.6 ± 3.9	69.5 ± 3.0
	ML	45.1 ± 4.5	47.9 ± 4.2	42.2 ± 2.9
	MW	30.4 ± 3.0	32.8 ± 2.1	28.1 ± 1.4
Femur	FCW	78.7 ± 6.7	84.2 ± 4.3	73.4 ± 3.6
	FL	52.2 ± 4.9	54.3 ± 4.8	50.2 ± 4.1
	FW	28.9 ± 3.3	30.6 ± 3.4	27.3 ± 2.6

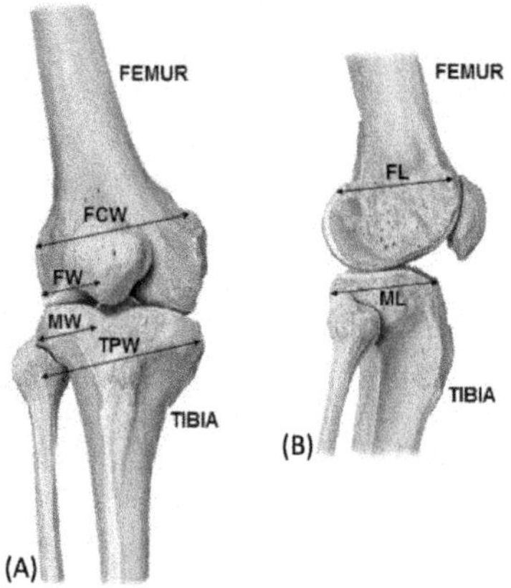

FIGURE 6.1
Knee bones dimensions, (A) anterior and (B) lateral view [10]: Femur Condyle Width (FCW), medial Femur Width (FW), tibial plateau Medial Width (MW), Tibial Plateau Width (TPW), medial Femoral condyle Length (FL), and tibial plateau Medial Length (ML).

male subjects are about 13 % – 15 % higher than in female ones, as shown in Tab. 6.1.

In order to facilitate fluid bending/straightening motions and to protect the joint against weight-bearing stresses, as well as to reduce the internal friction in the joint, all articular surfaces are covered with cartilage, a special protective and flexible connective tissue. The synovial fluid is the thick liquid that lubricates joints and keeps them moving smoothly. The knee joint is enclosed by a joint capsule, with four sturdy ligaments: two collateral ligaments placed along the sides of the knee that gives stability to the knee, limiting the sideways motion. Instead, two cruciate ligaments, crossing within the joint,

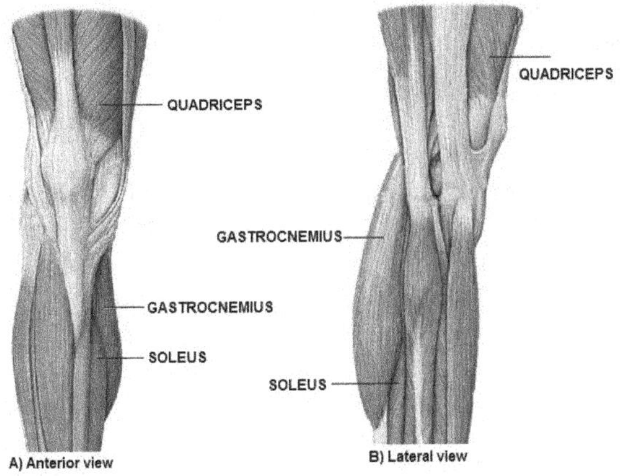

FIGURE 6.2
Example of knee muscles: A) anterior view and B) lateral view [10].

connects the tibia to the femur for controlling rotation, forward and backward movements of the tibia [185, 186].

Despite the numerous anatomical structures that compose the knee joint, such as synovial fluid, bursa, minor ligaments, tendons, that guarantee the stability and functionality of the joint [187], only the most important, the femur, tibia-patella, will be considered in the knee model illustrated in the following sections.

6.2.1 Dielectric Properties

The dielectric properties of biological materials represent a measure of their response to an applied electric field. The electric field and the biological tissues interact at all levels, from the cellular to the molecular level, and their interaction induces conduction and polarization currents within biological systems.

The structure and composition of biological tissues establish the nature and sort of their interaction with electromagnetic fields, and the resulting dielectric spectrum. However, tissues can be modelled as dielectric materials characterized by polarization mechanisms and dielectric losses.

When an external sinusoidal field excites the tissue, the electrical charges displacements generate polarization mechanisms. The dielectric losses arise from conduction currents inside the tissue together with the lossy effects caused by the material polarization. The physical parameter associated with this phenomenon is the electrical conductivity, whose continuous component accounts the polarization of the bound charges, while the alternate components accounts the energy losses due to bound charges and dipole relaxations.

Dielectric properties of biological tissues in the frequency domain are described by a complex and frequency-dependent dielectric function: the electrical permittivity, an intrinsic property of dielectric materials. In dealing with tissues, the dielectric properties are the frequency variations of the relative permittivity and the electrical conductivity, as reported over years by various investigators [13]. The main characteristics of the dielectric frequency properties of biological tissues consist of three main relaxation regions. Each of them is characterized by a specific polarization mechanism, namely α, β, and γ regions, respectively at low, medium, and high frequency, and other minor dispersion, such as the often reported δ dispersion.

Several models were used to describe tissue electrical biological behaviour. However, the model built on the expressions provided by Cole-Cole is even nowadays one of the most widely employed. The Cole-Cole equation describes the relaxation phenomena in dielectrics, and represents a modification of the Debye relaxation. The following expresses the effective dielectric permittivity [188]:

$$\dot{\varepsilon}_{eff}(\omega) = \varepsilon_\infty + \sum_n \frac{\Delta\varepsilon_n}{1 + (j\omega\tau_n)^{1-\alpha_n}} + \frac{\sigma_{dc}}{j\omega\varepsilon_0} \tag{6.1}$$

where:

- ε_∞ namely, the infinite permittivity, is the value of permittivity in high-frequency range, where the dielectric can be considered as unrelaxed;
- ε_0 is the permittivity of free space;
- $\Delta\varepsilon_n$ is the magnitude of the dispersion described as difference between ε_s known as static permittivity, and ε_∞ in relation to the n-th relaxation phenomenon;
- τ_n is the relaxation time of the n-th relaxation phenomenon, that is the necessary time for dipoles to return into a relaxed state after the perturbation by an electromagnetic field;
- ω is the angular frequency;
- α_n is an empiric coefficient affecting the spectral frequency shape of the n-th relaxation phenomenon; in particular, its range is $0 < \alpha_n < 1$ and the higher its value, the higher the flattening of the spectrum;
- and σ_{dc} is the static conductivity.

Several studies investigated the electrical characterization of human biological tissues, ranging from skin, fat, muscles and bones. Tab. 6.3 summarizes some of the most extensive and detailed electrical characterization works of biological tissues [189–191]. However, as far as we know, no specific in-vivo studies have ever been conducted to characterize human knee electrical behaviour.

6.3 Knee Model

In this section, the realization of a personalized model of human knee is illustrated. The subject-specific finite element modelling allows the optimization of electrodes design and adhesion, as well as a better understanding of the of human body behaviour by evaluating the injuries extent and therapeutics treatments progress. In Chapter 9, the human knee model, here illustrated, will be applied to enhance the inter-individual reproducibility of a measurement method for monitoring NSAIDs after transdermal delivery in clinical practice.

The *Generic Model* (Fig. 6.3) is based on the solution of Maxwell Equations in the electric-quasistationary limit via Finite Element Analysis. They interact with the *Geometry Equations* on the basis of the Default Settings which account for Geometric and Tissues Dielectric Properties. The Personalized Model can be generated by exploiting as input individual data (knee circumference at the patella, body mass index, and sex of the specific patient), realizing thus the *Layers Thickness Customization.* Moreover, by means of impedance spectroscopy measurements, performed before the drug administration, a *Dielectric Parameters Customization* is performed.

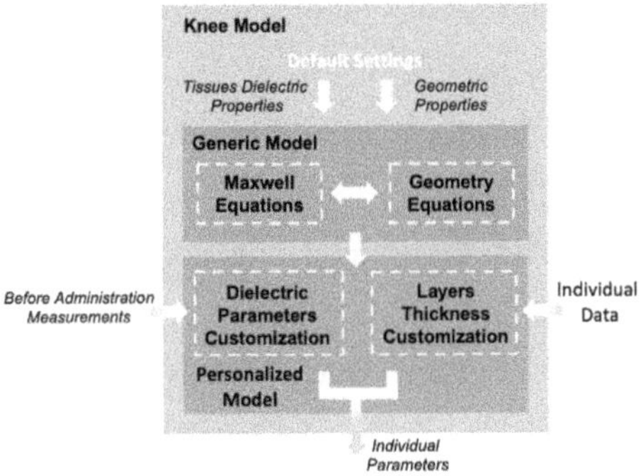

FIGURE 6.3
Personalized FEM model of the human knee.

6.3.1 Geometry Modelling

Finite element analysis (FEA) is a powerful tool for evaluating questions of functional morphology, for the numerical analysis of the biomechanical behaviour of human body's structures, to solve problems in orthopaedics, as well as to model soft tissue structures throughout the human body. Under the best of circumstances, FEA is a non-trivial task, since it requires plenty of time and specific parameters to develop the required model representation of the system to be modelled, especially if it is human.

Three categories of input data are needed to appropriately implement FEA; they include material properties, boundary conditions, and geometry, that is, the size and shape of the object of interest.

The simplified knee structure, presented in this section, consists of the femur-tibia-patella articulation enclosed into a multi-layered cylinder modelling different tissues, i.e., Muscle, Subcutaneous Fat and Skin listed from innermost to outermost layer. The skin is the outermost layer of the knee; it is a keratinized multi-layered epithelial tissue, consisting of many sub-layers with different biological characteristics and thickness [192]. The outermost skin layer is the epidermis, with thickness ranging between 20 μm to 300 μm [193]. It is composed by different substrates, namely, stratum corneum, lucidum, granulosum, spinosum, and basale [194]. Then, the dermis with thickness ranging between 1 mm to 7 mm, occurs, and it varies in male and female [192,195]. Then, we have hypodermis with subcutaneous adipose tissue, where the Subcutaneous Fat Thickness (SFT) depends on the body district, the sex, and the physical subject conditions, as well as the skin thickness [195,196]. In this model, according to the different amount of water, which varies significantly from the stratum corneum to dermis [23,197,198].

The skin layers have been arranged into two main sub-layers, namely Wet and Dry skin. In what follows, the cylindrical model with five layers is stated.

- *Layer 1*: it models the outermost part of the skin i.e., stratum corneum and lucidum, namely *Dry Skin*;
- *Layer 2*: it includes stratum granulosum, spinosum, basale, and dermis, namely *Wet Skin*;
- *Layer 3*: it includes the innermost part hypoderm, subcutaneous fat tissue, namely *SFT*;
- *Layer 4*: muscle;
- *Layer 5*: bone.

Fig. 6.4 shows a sketches of the geometrical structure of the knee articulation and tissues layering.

In Tab. 6.2, an example of model layers thickness [mm] both for male and females is reported, by assuming mean radius of knee circumference equal to 6.5 cm and Body Mass Index (BMI) equal to 23 kg\m^2.

Since physical parameters vary greatly among different subjects, an algorithm able to calculate personalized thicknesses of the five layers is to be introduced. The considered input parameters are the sex, the Body Mass Index (BMI) and the radius of the mean circumference of knee (mean-radius). BMI is an indicator of body composition and it is generally calculated as person's weight in kilograms divided by the square of height in meters. The radius is obtained by measuring the knee in three different points, in detail at the centre of patella and 5 cm above and below this latter.

The algorithm consists of the following steps:

- definition of *Layer 5* and *Layer 2* thicknesses based on sex, according to Tabs. 6.1 and 6.2;
- application of the linear relation [199] to calculate the thickness of *Layer 3* (SFT):

$$BMI = 0.385SFT + 16.991; \tag{6.2}$$

- and computation of the thickness of *Layer 4* as the difference between the *mean-radius* and the thicknesses of other layers, having constrained *Layer 1* at 60 μm both for males and females [193, 200, 201].

.

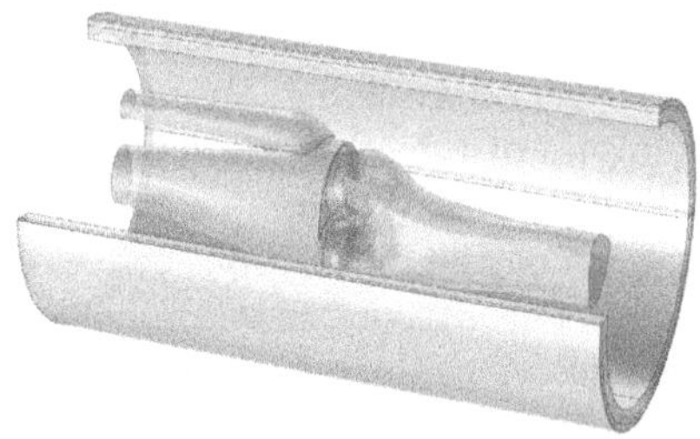

FIGURE 6.4
3D model of human knee [11].

TABLE 6.2
Thicknesses [mm] of model layers for males and females (BMI = of 23 kg\m^2, and radius of mean circumference = 6.5 cm).

	Layer 1: Dry Skin	**Layer 2:** Wet Skin	**Layer 3:** Fat	**Layer 4:** Muscle	**Layer 5:** Bone
Male	0.060	4.501	15.192	15.621	25.640
Female	0.060	3.666	16.971	17.552	22.760

6.3.2 Dielectric Modelling

All the above-mentioned different tissues are represented by a unique dielectric function, with the exception of muscles. The electrical parameters, listed in Tab 6.3, represent the inputs of the knee model, which will subsequently be optimized and customized.

The muscles of knee joint are skeletal muscles, which are attached to the skeleton by tendons in order to control the voluntary movements of the body. The skeletal muscles are tissues composed by fibers organized into bundles, called fascicles, surrounded by a middle layer of connective tissue. The muscle fibers are reciprocally parallel, whereas the fascicle can be characterized by variable directions (they may also differ from tendons direction) [202]. Therefore, the skeletal muscle has anisotropic properties according to the muscle fibers direction (Fig. 6.2) [203–205]. As widely confirmed by scientific literature, the muscles show different dielectric properties depending on the direction (perpendicular and along) of their fibers. Indeed, several frequency ranges are reported in [131] for the imaginary and real component of the Effective Dielectric Permittivity. However, both the values and expression of the Effective Dielectric Permittivity of all knee tissues are reported in literature, with the exception of muscles. Indeed, for knee muscles only the dielectric description, corresponding to the application of an external excitation field perpendicular to the muscle fibers direction, is available. By means of an identification procedure, based on the samples of Effective Dielectric Permittivity function presented in [131], a more comprehensive muscular model is implemented.

This model takes into account the anisotropic behaviour of the muscles. The scalar Effective Dielectric Permittivity function is expressed as a diagonal anisotropic tensor, which describes the muscular electrical behaviour when the muscle is subjected to an external electric field along whatever direction. The main purpose of this procedure is to identify all the parameters of the Cole-Cole equation (6.1), which describes the behaviour of the muscle, excited along the fibers, in order to allow the fitting of both imaginary and real parts of its Effective Dielectric Permittivity frequency spectra, to the data experimentally obtained by Gabriel in [131]. This is expressed as a constraint in the identification problem imposed in order to minimize the distance between the aforementioned unknown parameters and the parameters of the muscle excited along the perpendicular direction of the fibers. Consequently, the identification issue is settled as:

$$\min \| \underline{x}_{LD} - \underline{x}_{TD} \| \tag{6.3}$$

subject to:

$$\dot{\varepsilon}_{eff}(\omega_k, \underline{x}_{LD}) - \dot{\varepsilon}_{eff_{exp}}(\omega_k) = 0 \tag{6.4}$$

where:

- $\underline{x}_{LD}$ represents the Cole-Cole parameters vector of the Effective Dielectric Permittivity when the specific tissue is stimulated by an electric field along the fibers direction,

TABLE 6.3
Parameters of Cole-Cole equation according to Eq. (6.3) for Muscles P. (Parallel) and according to [13] for other biological tissue.

	ε_∞	$\Delta\varepsilon_1$	τ_1 [ps]	α_1	$\Delta\varepsilon_2$	τ_2 [ns]	α_2	$\Delta\varepsilon_3$	τ_3 [μs]	α_3	$\Delta\varepsilon_4$	τ_4 [ms]	α_4	σ_{dc} [S/m]
Dry Skin	4.0	32.0	7.23	0.00	1100	32.48	0.00							0.0002
Wet Skin	4.0	39.0	7.96	0.10	280	79.58	0.00	3.0×10^4	1.59	0.16	3.0×10^4	1.592	0.20	0.0004
Fat	2.5	9.0	7.96	0.20	35	15.92	0.10	3.3×10^4	159.15	0.05	1.0×10^7	15.915	0.01	0.0350
Muscle T.	4.0	50.0	7.23	0.10	7000	353.68	0.10	1.2×10^6	318.31	0.10	2.5×10^7	2.274	0.00	0.2000
Muscle P.	4.0	50.0	10.57	0.11	7000	19.10	0.01	1.2×10^6	725.47	0.32	2.5×10^7	0.737	0.00	0.2397
Bone	2.5	18.0	13.26	0.22	300	79.58	0.25	2×10^4	159.15	0.20	2.0×10^7	15.915	0.00	0.0700

- $\underline{x}_{TD}$ represents the Cole-Cole parameters vector of the Effective Dielectric Permittivity when the specific tissue is stimulated by an electric field perpendicular to the fibers direction,
- and ω_k represents the sampling frequency of the experimental data.

The complex equality limitation is described by a nonlinear function of degrees of freedom. The issue is specified as a convex optimization problem and its solution is obtained through the Interior-Point optimization procedure. The solution quality is assessed as prediction error in the experimental data fitting:

$$\varepsilon_{fit_{re}} = \frac{\|\mathfrak{Re}\{\dot{\varepsilon}_{eff_{fit}}(\omega_k, \underline{x}_{LD}) - \dot{\varepsilon}_{eff_{exp}}(\omega_k)\}\|}{\|\mathfrak{Re}\{\dot{\varepsilon}_{eff_{exp}}(\omega_k)\}\|} \tag{6.5}$$

$$\varepsilon_{fit_{im}} = \frac{\|\mathfrak{Im}\{\dot{\varepsilon}_{eff_{fit}}(\omega_k, \underline{x}_{LD}) - \dot{\varepsilon}_{eff_{exp}}(\omega_k)\}\|}{\|\mathfrak{Im}\{\dot{\varepsilon}_{eff_{exp}}(\omega_k)\}\|} \tag{6.6}$$

the fitted Effective Dielectric Permittivity is sampled at experimental frequency both for its simulated real and the imaginary part. By means of this procedure, the Cole-Cole equation parameters can be determined with a prediction error lower than 10 % on the reconstruction of the $\dot{\varepsilon}_{eff}(\omega)$ real part, and lower than 5 % on the reconstruction of its imaginary part. The results, in terms of fitting, achieved in relation to both the dielectric permittivity and the equivalent conductivity frequency spectra are shown in Fig. 6.5.

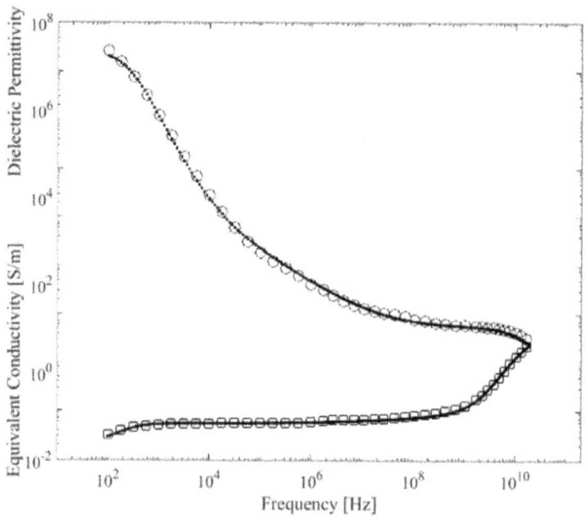

FIGURE 6.5
Experimental (circles) and fitted (dotted line) dielectric permittivity with experimental (squares) and fitted (solid line) equivalent conductivity of muscles (excitation parallel to fibers).

The Cole-Cole parameters values, along with the same values characteristics of other tissues included in the presented knee joint model, are reported in Tab. 6.3.

6.3.3 Electric Differential Model

The presented numerical human knee model relies on the Finite Element Analysis of Partial Differential Equations obtained by considering the Direct Current Maxwell equation in the frequency domain and the lossy dielectric materials characterized by relaxation phenomena. Furthermore, Maxwell equations can be simplified into the quasi-stationary electrical limit, by neglecting the time derivative of the flux density field, and by considering simultaneously both the current density filed into the tissues and the curl-free electric field. About the current density, the contribution of the external current has been neglected, owing to the voltage-driven excitation; therefore, current density is represented by two main contributions: Maxwell displacement current corresponding to the displacement field variation rate, and the conduction current produced by ohmic conduction. The unknown scalar field of the differential problem in Eq. (6.7), a general formulation, which consider the dielectric transfer function in terms of its effective dielectric permittivity, is the scalar electric potential:

$$\begin{cases} -\varepsilon_0 \dot{\varepsilon} \nabla^2 \overline{\varphi} + \nabla \cdot \overline{J}_{ext} = 0 \\ \overline{\varphi}|_{\partial\Omega_T} = \overline{\varphi}_0(\mathbf{r}) \\ -\sigma_{dc} \nabla \overline{\varphi} \cdot \hat{n}|_{\partial\Omega_S} = J_n(\mathbf{r}) \end{cases} \tag{6.7}$$

where:

- $\overline{\varphi}$ represents the phasor of electric scalar potential;
- $\overline{\varphi}_0(\mathbf{r})$ is the Dirichlet boundary condition value set on the boundary $\partial\Omega_T$;
- and $\overline{J}_n(\mathbf{r})$ is the Neumann boundary condition value set on the boundary $\partial\Omega_S$.

The normal component value of the total current across the surfaces is imposed by Neumann boundary condition. The electric scalar potential value across the voltage source terminals, namely Ω_T, is imposed by Dirichlet boundary condition. Specifically, the Neumann boundary condition sets a natural global boundary condition (i.e., electric insulation) on the skin surface Ω_S.

Finally, the equations in (6.7) must be coupled with appropriate conditions set at the interface between two distinct tissues, by affirming the continuity of the current density normal component field along the separation surface.

Part III

Case Studies

7

Aesthetics Medicine

CONTENTS

This chapter illustrates the application of the instrument DUSM, presented in Chapter 3, to the non-invasive assessment of the drug under the skin during aesthetics treatments. Therefore, three experimental campaigns, based on impedance spectroscopy of the biological tissue, are described: (*i*) in-vitro laboratory emulations on eggplants, (*ii*) ex-vivo tests on pig ears, and ultimately (*iii*) in-vivo tests on human volunteers. The results confirm the appropriateness of impedance measurement for assessing the amount of drug penetrated into the skin after transdermal delivery with reasonable metrological performance.

7.1 In-vitro Metrological Characterization of the DUSM

The feasibility of a method for assessing non-invasively the drug under the skin, based on impedance spectroscopy, was proven in Chapter 2. In this section, the DUSM, described and characterized in Chapter 3, is tested metrologically by referring to its typical use in aesthetic treatments.

In fact, for in-vivo metrological characterization, the physician injects a water soluble sodium salt of hyaluronic acid for the patient treatment. The hyaluronic acid injections, well known as dermal fillers, are becoming increasingly popular for aesthetic treatments. Hyaluronic acid is a disaccharide naturally present in all human connective tissues, including the skin. This molecule is essential for collagen matrix and elastic fiber formation, as well as for

DOI: 10.1201/9781003170143-7

increasing skin moisture levels and accelerating regeneration and healing. These injections have become an essential part of aesthetic treatments, such as facial rejuvenation or harmonization. In particular, they are used to correct disharmonies by restoring lost skin volume, together with modification of congenital characteristics and reduction of the appearance of unwanted wrinkles and lines.

Preliminary tests are conducted on eggplants and pig ears for analyzing different parameters, i.e., short-term stability (10 min), sensitivity at varying the delivered drug, and reproducibility over biological tissues.

One of the most important aspects to take into account for the experimental planning of calibration is the measurement reference. Thus, a calibrated syringe is used to deposit a reference drug volume in the tissue. A known volume of drug, delivered by injection at a fixed depth, is used as metrological reference for the characterization.

Actually, injection of drug into the skin cannot be properly considered as a transdermal delivery. However, regardless of the kinetics that led the drug into the tissue, the calibrated syringe ensures a reference amount of drug actually present by a resolution compatible with a treatment based on transdermal delivery. In other terms, the calibrated syringe is used only for emulating the transdermal delivery for metrological purposes.

7.1.1 Experimental Setup

Ten eggplants, able to emulate the electrical behaviour of human skin, are peeled and dried, then cut as parallelepipeds of size 40 mm × 40 mm × 30 mm (Fig. 7.1).

On the eggplants samples, pre-gelled electrodes PG500FIAB 28 mm × 36 mm are longitudinally cut in half 14 mm × 36 mm and placed on the samples surface at a distance of 1 cm (Fig. 7.1). A sinusoidal signal with an amplitude of 100 mV is applied by the DUSM, while the frequency varied on a logarithmic scale from 0.1 Hz to 49.0 kHz.

7.1.2 Short-term Stability

Unwanted effects are minimized and the device configuration is optimized by investigating the influence of the input frequency on the metrological performance during 600 s.

Stability is a property of a measuring instrument, representing the aptitude of an instrument to provide measurements values that are mutually slightly different, in consecutive measurements taken independently of the same measurand, in a defined time interval, with a unified procedure, by the same operator, under the same conditions for the influence quantities [152].

Procedure. On all the eggplants samples, eleven electrical impedance spectra, each 60 s, are recorded in 10 min. All the tests are carried out without injecting drug in the eggplants, with the goal of evaluating the influence of

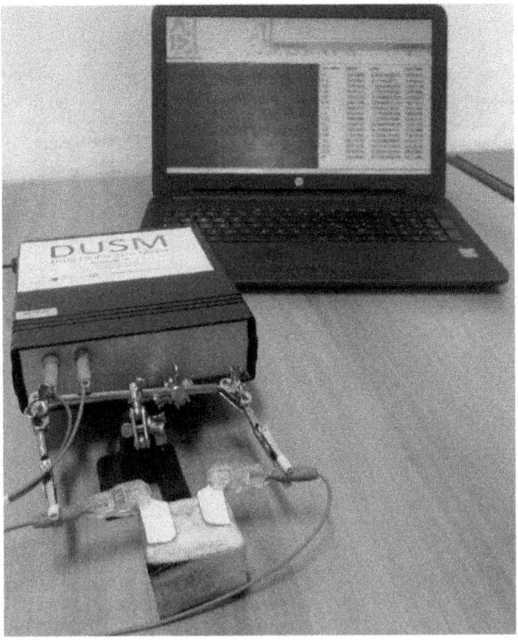

FIGURE 7.1
In-vitro test setup on eggplant pulp.

the electrode gel (progressively penetrating the tissue) on the measurements, in the range 0.1 Hz to 49.0 kHz.

For each frequency, stability is computed as the standard deviation among the 11 impedance values, measured during the 10-min test on a single eggplant sample. Then, the average stability is assessed on 10 samples at a fixed frequency. Finally, the overall average percentage stability is calculated over the frequency bandwidth as a whole.

Results. The average percentage short-term stability in relation to frequency plot is shown in Fig. 7.2 for the impedance magnitude. According to the preliminary experimental campaign results, the phase is not considered in this study. At 1.0 kHz, a deviation of 0.5 % is experienced, lower than at 14.2 kHz.

Accordingly, 1.0 kHz is confirmed as the working frequency with the aim of maximizing short-term stability.

7.1.3 Sensitivity

According to the VIM definition, the sensitivity represents the "quotient of the change in an indication of a measuring system and the corresponding change in a value of a quantity being measured" [152]. In the practice, it can

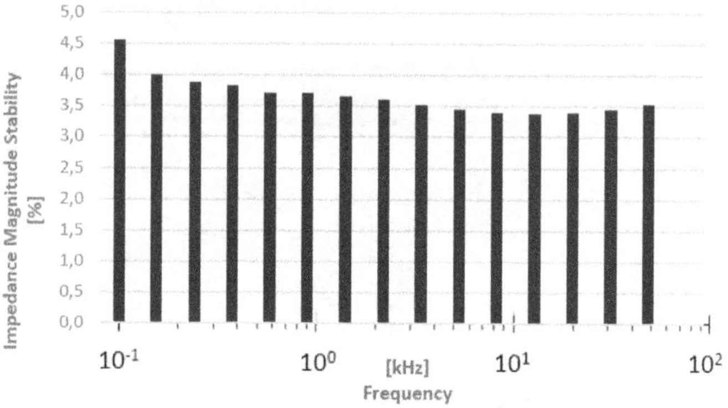

FIGURE 7.2
Average percentage 10-min stability of impedance magnitude vs operating frequency [4].

be assessed as the inverse of the slope in one point of the calibration curve. The sensitivity is mainly affected by the conductivity of the drug.

For evaluating the sensitivity, an experimental campaign is carried out at varying the injected solution conductivity and its principal influence parameters. For this purpose, a generic drug is modelled as a solution of an active principle (solute) in an aqueous excipient (solvent).

Main factors influencing the solution conductivity can be summarized as [206]: (i) *type of solution*, mainly expressed as viscosity and polarity in impedance spectroscopy; and (ii) *type and concentration of the solute*, mainly expressed as dissociation degree, ionic charge, and mobility, where the solute is defined electrochemically.

However, owing to the poor reliability of biological tissues models represented by a dense solution of cells, the relationship between these parameters and the system sensitivity cannot be determined with analytic methods. In fact, such models present influence parameters not sufficiently investigated to date [193].

For this reason, an a-posteriori black-box modelling approach, based on statistical Design of Experiments (DoE) [155], is adopted. DoE is an effective statistical and mathematical method for planning experiments in order to obtain data that once analyzed can yield valid and objective conclusions.

The first step of DoE is determining the objectives of an experiment and selecting the process factors for the study. Among the different kinds of DoE, the Taguchi experimental plan, already presented in Chapter 2, has been adopted. Thus, intentional changes are made to the controllable parameters in order to observe the corresponding changes in the output response.

In particular, the solution viscosity and solute concentration are experimented, owing to their independent and opposite influence on the solution conductivity, and therefore, on the device sensitivity. In the experiments, the solution viscosity was varied by adding sucrose ($C_{12}H_{22}O_{11}$) to demineralized water as a thickener, in order to achieve three molality levels: 0.00 mol/kg, 0.42 mol/kg, and 0.89 mol/kg. As solute, an electrolyte, and namely the sodium chloride $NaCl$, is experimented for its capability of ionic dissociation. In particular, the following molality levels are selected: 1.20 mol/kg, 2.40 mol/kg, and 3.60 mol/kg. Therefore, the experimental models were [155],

- for the *solution conductivity* γ:

$$\gamma = \sum_{j=1}^{n} (\alpha_{1j} + \alpha_{2j}) + u \tag{7.1}$$

  where α_{1j} and α_{2j} are the effects of the concentrations of thickener and solute, respectively, at the j-th level, on the solution conductivity, and u is the model uncertainty;

- for the *device sensitivity* β:

$$\beta = \sum_{j=1}^{n} (\delta_{1j} + \delta_{2j}) + u \tag{7.2}$$

  where δ_{1j} and δ_{2j} are the effects of the concentrations of thickener and solute, respectively, at the j-th level, on the device sensitivity.

The models are identified by the two-parameter three-level experimental plan L9 (factorial plan 3^2) [207] of Tab. 7.1.

The nine different solutions are injected in nine different eggplants. Each solution, injected in a sample of a specific eggplant, is delivered in five consecutive constant volume steps: 0.05 ml, 0.10 ml, 0.15 ml, 0.20 ml, and 0.25 ml. On the eggplants, the electrodes are placed at a distance of 2.0 cm and their area is 3.64 cm^2. The penetration depth of the needle is 2.5 cm.

In each experiment, a sinusoidal voltage with amplitude 100 mV and frequency 1 kHz is applied. The percentage variation from the initial impedance magnitude for all the volumes injected in the eggplant pulp is measured. For each experiment, the measurement is repeated 60 times; in particular, 10 for each of the 6 levels of injected solution. The first measurement is carried out without any injected solution, while the following 5 steps with the solution injection.

The sensitivity [ml^{-1}] is computed as the slope of the linear regression of the measured relative impedance mean over the injected volume.

Results of both solution conductivity and sensitivity are shown in the last two columns on the right of Tab. 7.1, respectively. Through the above results, the models coefficients α_{ij} and δ_{ij} are determined by the Analysis of Mean (ANOM) [157]. The coefficients are reported in Figs. 7.3 (a) and (b), respectively. In the same figures, the 1-σ uncertainty, determined by the Analysis of Variance (ANOVA), is highlighted.

TABLE 7.1
Two-parameter three-level experimental plan L9 (factorial plan 3^2) for testing sensitivity at varying delivered drug characteristics.

	Parameters		Results	
Run	Thickener concentration [mol/kg]	Electrolyte concentration [mol/kg]	Solution conductivity [$S \cdot 10^{-1} \cdot cm^{-1}$]	Device sensitivity [ml^{-1}]
1	0.00	1.20	1.08	140.66
2	0.00	2.40	1.43	66.98
3	0.00	3.60	1.66	110.16
4	0.42	1.20	0.87	84.94
5	0.42	2.40	1.23	85.91
6	0.42	3.60	1.41	112.01
7	0.98	1.20	0.50	66.94
8	0.98	2.40	0.87	72.02
9	0.98	3.60	1.09	133.67

The effects of the solution viscosity (thickener concentration) α_{1j} and the electrolyte solute concentration α_{2j} on the solution conductivity γ (Fig. 7.3 (a)) are mutually balanced: they decrease and grow, respectively, monotonously. The effects on device sensitivity β are quite different (Fig. 7.3 (b)).

ANOVA highlights a negligible effect of the solution viscosity (Fig. 7.3b, left), with a Variance Ratio of 0.24. The corresponding effects α_{1j} are included into the model uncertainty (*pooling error* method [207]), by increasing the statistical significance of the electrolyte concentration (Variance Ratio of 2.46). Furthermore, a non-monotonous trend of the electrolyte effect is highlighted (Fig. 2.10b, right).

In any case, a strong level of uncertainty affects the model (Fig. 7.3) of β. This arises mainly from the lack of inter- and intra-individual reproducibility of the eggplant in emulating biological tissue.

Finally, this study highlights the need for further investigation on other chemical parameters, such as ionic charge, charge/beam ratio, mass, ion-ion interaction forces, ion-solvent interaction forces, and so on, for future clinical application. As a matter of fact, the only electrical conductivity of the solution may be not sufficient for characterizing the measurement sensitivity.

7.1.4 Reproducibility

The reproducibility of an experiment refers to a set of measurement conditions that includes different locations, operators, measuring systems, and replicate measurements on the same or similar objects. Technically, the reproducibility

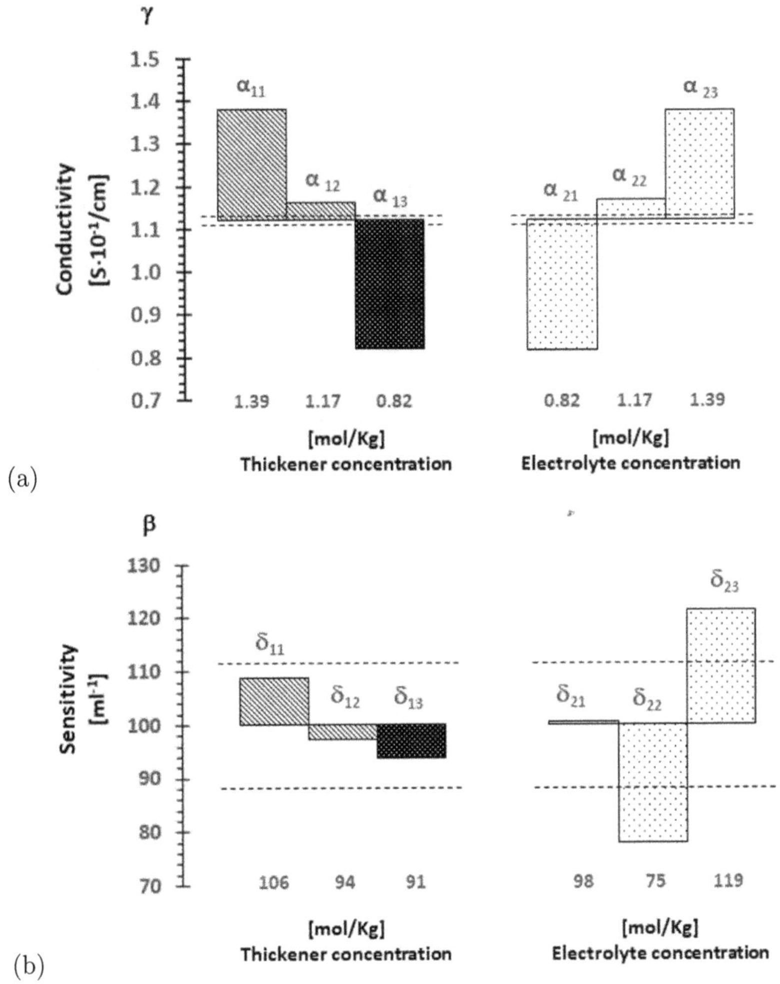

FIGURE 7.3
Influence of solution viscosity and solute concentration on (a) solution conductivity γ and (b) sensitivity β (dashed line: 1-σ model uncertainty) [4].

is the capability of an experiment to obtain consistent measures when the procedure is carried out in a different context (homologues devices, different laboratory, or operator). It can be considered as a characteristic of an experiment, meaning its aptitude to provide slightly dispersed measures in different conditions [152].

In this experiment, the inter- and intra-individual reproducibility are tested on different eggplants, as well as on a same eggplant using different parts.

Reproducibility is assessed as the standard deviation of impedance results over 10 eggplant samples, measured at a specific frequency, and at a given time elapsed from electrode application.

Results of Fig. 7.4 show how an increase in standard deviation, with respect the initial value, more than 300 %, after 10 min from electrode application. In particular, at 1.0 kHz (the most common working frequency in literature), the deviation from the minimum recorded at 14.2 kHz is less than 0.5 %.

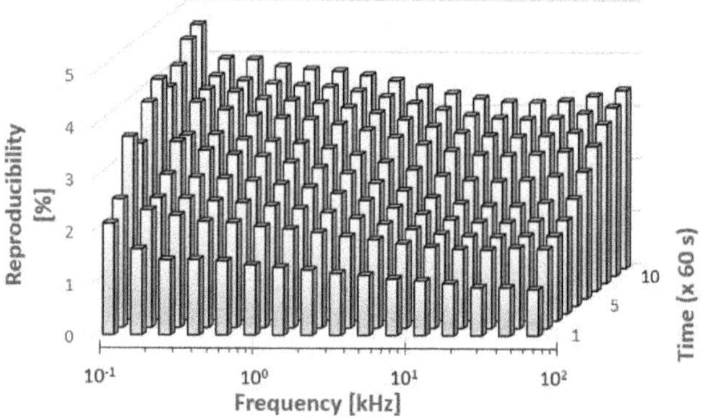

FIGURE 7.4
Reproducibility, assessed as standard deviation of impedance magnitude percentage variation with respect to initial value, over 10 eggplant samples, vs time and frequency [4].

7.2 Ex-vivo Metrological Characterization

In ex-vivo tests, a standard sterile syringe is used to calibrate the DUSM, owing to its possibility to inject a known amount of drug in the tissue under test.

In the following experiments, animal tissues are used to emulate the electrical behaviour of the human skin. Electrical impedance of biological materials is a complex quantity, which depends on the frequency and amplitude of the applied ac signal. It also depends on the tissue composition defined by the cells membranes and their protein-lipid-protein structure, as well as, extra and intra-cellular fluid. As a result, animal tissues, owing to their complex physiological and physiochemical structures, show a variable response over a wide band of signal frequency. Hence, they are suitably used in electrical impedance spectroscopy studies, conducted over a broad range of signal frequency using impedance analyzers.

According to well-established literature [158, 159], porcine skin is often used to evaluate topical and transdermal drug delivery, either in vivo, and in vitro. The use of porcine skin is broadly recognized due to ready availability and affordable cost, but most of all, the epidermal thickness and the lipid composition, as well as membrane permeability to diverse compounds, are significantly similar to human skin [160].

Eight pig ears are bought in a local abattoir, to preserve the tissue until the experimental procedure, and stored at 4 °C. The experiments are performed the same day, since it has been established that the maximum *post-mortem* time cell viability is not significantly reduced before 24 h at 4 °C [208]. The pig skin surface is cleaned and dried, then dead cells of the stratum corneum are removed by stripping an adhesive tape of 5 cm × 5 cm placed on the surface, 20 times by a single movement (Fig. 7.5). The tape stripping is widely used in ex-vivo and in-vivo studies to enhance measurement reproducibility [27, 142]. In these ex-vivo experiments, tape stripping is only a laboratory expedient to improve measurement quality, typical in metrological practice, however, in in-vivo use, only a mild cleansing is sufficient.

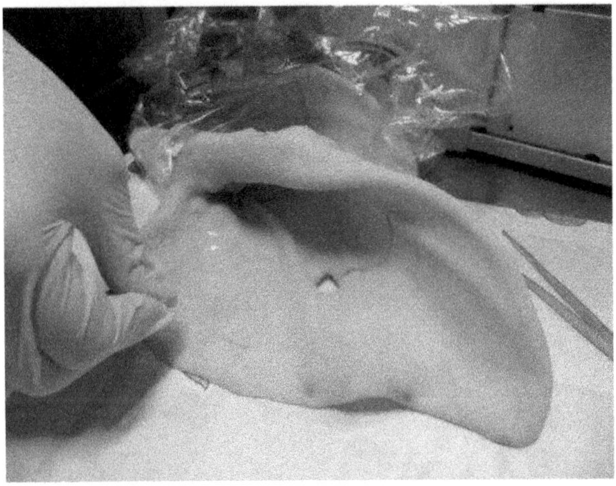

FIGURE 7.5
Laboratory test on pig ear [4].

A solution of hyaluronic acid sodium salt in saline water, with conductivity of 1.37 mS/cm, is injected 0.5 cm below the skin surface by the calibrated syringe. The measurement conditions are summarized in Tab. 7.2.

In particular, a sinusoidal constant current at 1 kHz frequency is imposed to the pig ear under test, through two identical square electrodes with surface

TABLE 7.2
Measurement conditions in ex-vivo metrological tests.

Signal Frequency	Electrodes Area	Electrodes Gap	Drug Conductivity
1.00 kHz	1.82 cm^2	1.4 cm	1.37 mS/cm

area of 1.82 cm^2 and distant from each other 1.4 cm. In this two-electrode method, used for studying the impedance variation, the current injection and voltage measurement are made using the same electrodes.

The experiments are repeated for 20 times by injecting the following solution volumes: 0.05 ml, 0.10 ml, 0.15 ml, 0.20 ml, and 0.25 ml, and by measuring the percentage variation from the initial impedance magnitude. For each injected volume, mean and standard deviation of percent impedance variation from initial value are assessed.

Percentage nonlinearity is computed by the analysis of variance (one-way ANOVA):

$$\sigma_{NL\%} = \sqrt{\sum_{k=1}^{n}(\hat{\epsilon}_k - \bar{\epsilon}_k)^2 \cdot \frac{1}{(n-1)}} \cdot \frac{100}{(y_{max} - y_{min})} \tag{7.3}$$

where n is the number of averaged experimental points, $\hat{\epsilon}_k$ is the k-th non linearity error, $\bar{\epsilon}_k$ the average linearity error, and y_{min} and y_{max} the lowest and highest level, respectively, of percentage impedance variation.

The resolution, defined as the smallest change in a quantity being measured that causes a perceptible change in the corresponding indication [152], here arises from the indeterminacy of the measured amount of drug, assessed by the uncertainty of a single point in the calibration curve again through one-way ANOVA:

$$\Delta_V = \sqrt{\frac{1}{\beta^2(n-2)}\left[\sum_{k=1}^{n}(y_k - \bar{y})^2 - \frac{\left[\sum_{k=1}^{n}(x_k - \bar{x})(y_k - \bar{y})\right]^2}{\sum_{k=1}^{n}(x_k - \bar{x})^2}\right]} \tag{7.4}$$

where β is the calibration curve angular coefficient, y_k and $\bar{y}_k$ the k-th and overall, respectively, averaged percentage impedance variation, and x_k and $\bar{x}_k$ the k-th and the average, properly, injected amount of drug.

The calibration curve expresses the relation between indication and corresponding measured quantity value, as a one-to-one relationship.

The calibration, under specified conditions, establishes a relationship between the quantity values with measurement uncertainties, provided by measurement standards, and the corresponding indications with associated measurement uncertainties.

Instrumental measurement uncertainty is obtained through calibration of a measuring instrument or measuring system, except for a primary measurement standard. In this case, a linear behaviour is experienced as pointed out in Fig. 7.6.

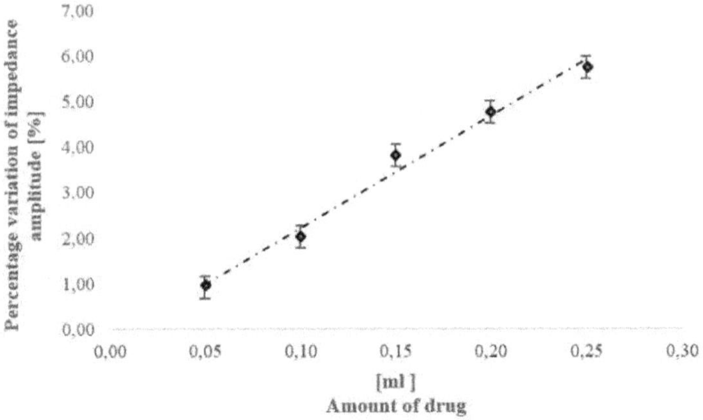

FIGURE 7.6
Percentage variation of impedance magnitude vs amount of drug in ex-vivo experiments [4].

The obtained sensitivity results [$ml^{-1} \cdot 10^{-1}$], 1-σ repeatability percentage [%], nonlinearity percentage [%], and resolution [ml] are shown in Tab. 7.3. The resolution is consistent with dermatological administration standards. The exploitation of substances with electrical conductivity higher than a few of mS/cm assure acceptable sensitivity: volumes of 10 ml of the tested solution achieve normalized impedance magnitude variations higher than 100 %.

Compared to the laboratory tests results, the repeatability decreases. As expected, the electrical response of animal cells is more unpredictable than the vegetable ones. The accuracy also degenerates due to the lower reproducibility implicit of ex-vivo tests.

The metrological characterization results of the prototyped DUSM highlight a resolution and sensitivity that make possible its use for in-vivo transdermal delivery in clinical application. De facto, the instrument proved its

TABLE 7.3
Metrological characteristics of the DUSM.

Sensitivity [$ml^{-1} \cdot 10^{-1}$]	1-σ Repeatability [%]	Nonlinearity [%]	Resolution [ml]
24.5	0.16	4.25	0.37

ability to assess the drug amount by measuring impedance spectrum before and after administration.

7.3 In-vivo Characterization

In-vivo testing is a vital aspect of medical research in general. In-vivo studies provide valuable information regarding the effects of a particular substance in a living organism.

For the DUSM, in-vivo experiments are carried out in an authorized Institute on subjects of different ages and sex (Fig. 7.7). The subjects gave their informed consent to participate to the study and the privacy consent to publish the related information, study results and images in scientific publications.

Drug injections are performed by a physician, while the measurements are carried out by means of DUSM, the instrument specifically prototyped for in-vivo use, in compliance with safety regulations, presented in the previous chapters [9]. All the measurements are carried out in accordance with relevant guidelines and regulations. In-vivo experimental tests follow the same

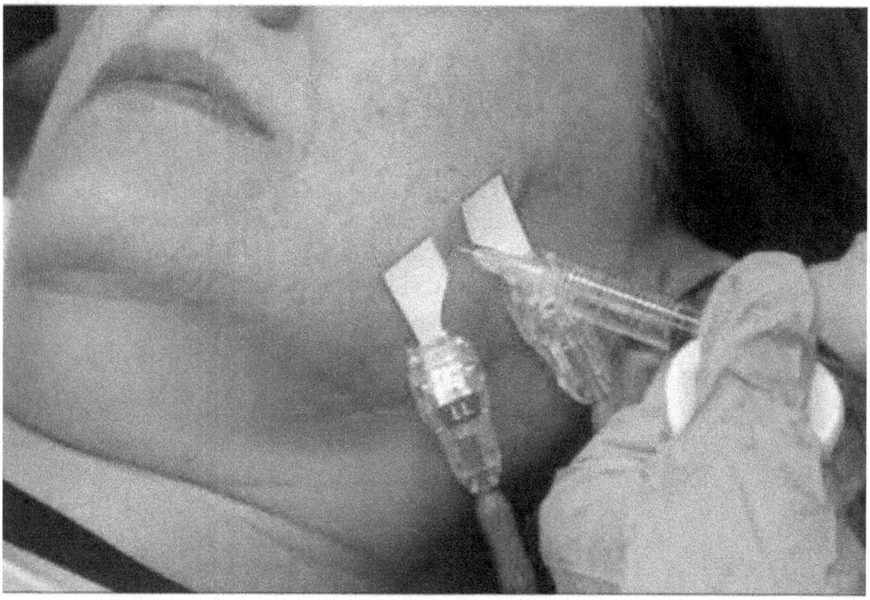

FIGURE 7.7
Drug injection during in-vivo experiments [2].

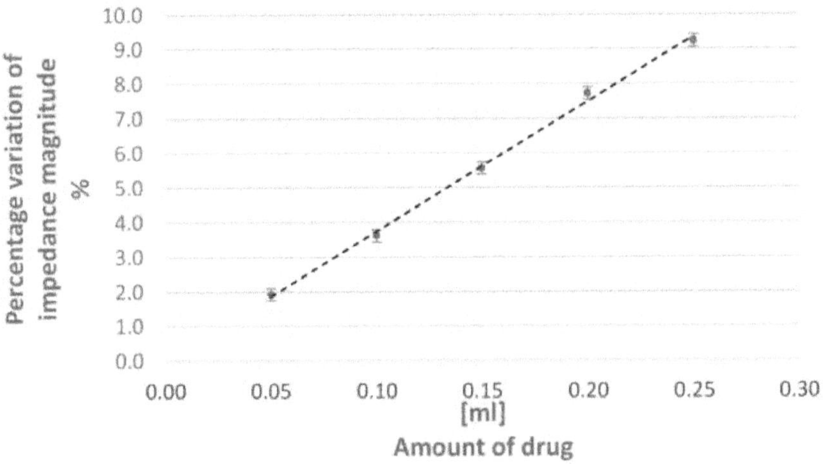

FIGURE 7.8
Impedance magnitude percentage variation vs drug amount in in-vivo experiments [2].

setup shown in the previous sections. The experimental tests point out that, for conditions equivalent to ex-vivo test, the setup design achieves maximum accuracy and repeatability in case of 520 mV stimulus signal level.

The solution injected is a water soluble sodium salt of hyaluronic acid, with conductivity of 1.37 mS/cm. It is injected 0.5 cm below the surface, such as in ordinary cosmetic treatments. The drug is injected in following successive volumes: 0.00 ml, 0.05 ml, 0.10 ml, 0.15 ml, 0.20 ml, and 0.25 ml and the experiments are repeated for 10 times on all 8 subjects. Meanwhile the measurement conditions include a drug with a conductivity of 1.37 mS/cm, a signal with and amplitude and frequency of 520 mV and 1.00 kHz respectively; and then, the electrodes surface of 1.82 cm^2 with an interelectrodes gap of 1.4 cm.

Also in this case, a linear behaviour between the percentage variation of the impedance magnitude and the amount of drug is found, as illustrated in Fig. 7.8.

7.3.1 Results Discussion

For the sake of the simplicity, in Tab. 7.4, the results of the method metrological characterization, presented in Chapter 2, are reported and compared to the results of the metrological characterization of the experimental

TABLE 7.4
Metrological characteristics of the assessment method in laboratory, ex-vivo, and in-vivo experiments.

	Sensitivity [ml^{-1}]	Nonlinearity [%]	1-σ Repeatability [%]	Accuracy [%]	Resolution [ml]
Laboratory experiments	29.5	2.35	0.07	5.23	0.23
Ex-vivo experiments	24.5	4.25	0.16	7.40	0.37
In-vivo experiments	22.7	3.31	0.27	5.71	0.19
Laboratory method	30.6	3.64	0.11	4.38	0.35
Ex-vivo method	34.4	5.04	0.47	6.20	0.44

campaigns presented above. In Tab. 7.4, in the first three rows, the metrological characteristics of in-vivo tests are compared with laboratory and ex-vivo performance. The same setup configuration, drug, and sample size are considered by using the DUSM instrument.

In summary, by comparing results of method metrological characterization and the ones obtained by DUSM, a comparable sensitivity can be observed. Although, the latter's decreases compared to values in Tab. 2.3 (last two rows), due to the higher viscosity of the solution injected in in-vivo tests.

By focusing on the experiments with the DUSM, despite different biological samples are used, namely, pig skin and eggplants, the obtained results are still comparable to those obtained in-vivo on human skin. In particular, by analyzing the three first rows, it follows:

- the nonlinearity is lower than in ex-vivo tests (3.31 % vs 4.25 %), although still lightly higher than in laboratory (2.35 %);
- the 1-σ repeatability is a little worse because it varies from 0.16 % to 0.27 % (though still again worse than in laboratory, 0.07 %);
- the accuracy improves from 7.40 % to 5.71 % and is still compatible with laboratory (5.23 %);
- the resolution improves from 0.37 ml to 0.19 ml, even higher than in laboratory (0.23 ml).

Such results highlight the suitability of impedance measurement for assessing the amount of drug actually penetrated into the skin after in-vivo treatment.

8

Diabetology

CONTENTS

This chapter illustrates the application of the Insulin Meter, presented in Chapter 5. The bioavailability is assessed non-invasively and in real-time after administration in clinical diabetology treatments. By means of local impedance measurements in the administration site, the bioavailability is assessed as the insulin decrease after the injection. A personalized model, i.e. customized to the specific subject, can be identified and validated during each insulin administration, by improving inter- and intra-individual reproducibility. Thus, three experimental campaigns with different setups, always based on impedance spectroscopy, are described: (i) in vitro on eggplants, (ii) ex vivo on pig abdominal non-perfused muscle, and ultimately, and (iii) in vivo on a human volunteer. In all the cases, subcutaneous injection is used as a reference of insulin. The experimental results highlight a better accuracy performance of the personalized model than a generic one.

8.1 In-vitro Metrological Characterization of the Insulin Meter

The feasibility of the measurement method underlying the Insulin Meter has been proven and illustrated in Chapter 4. In the following sections, the in-vitro, ex-vivo, and in-vivo tests are presented.

DOI: 10.1201/9781003170143-8

Experimentation is the best known way to test the veracity of scientific theories and to provide clues to causal inference. The first experimental tests of the Insulin Meter, detailed below, are conducted in vitro.

In-vitro tests are procedures or experiments, performed outside a living organism, in a controlled environment. This conditions allow to carry out more detailed analyses and to examine biological effects in a larger number of critical situations, than in animal or human trials. Therefore, also in this case, the experimental in-vitro campaign is conducted on eggplants, already shown as able to satisfyingly mimic the human tissues behaviour [145, 146].

In the following subsections, the tests for the drift, the sensitivity, the nonlinearity, the repeatability, the reproducibility, and the accuracy are illustrated. The results of each metrological characteristic are compared for both a generic and a personalized model.

Specifically, the generic model is identified off line during the metrological qualification tests on all the samples, such as it is common in traditional medicine. On the other hand, the personalized model is identified on line on the specific subject tissue, in definite measurement conditions. The generic model highlights the performance of the Insulin Meter applicable to every generic individual, but without taking into account the specific condition of the subject. Conversely, the personalized model highlights the performance specific to a single subject, and still valid in every use condition. In addition, two different configurations of the Insulin meter, namely two- and four-wire measurement, are tested and compared. Finally, for these two setup configurations, the differences in the parameters of greatest interest are pointed out.

8.1.1 Experimental Setup

In the in-vitro tests, the impedance intrinsic uncertainty, arising from water evaporation during the measurements, is mitigated by peeling ad drying the eggplants. In particular, they are dried for 2 h, in a controlled environment, at a temperature of 23 °C, and a relative humidity of 50 %. Each eggplant is cut in a rectangular block of 10 cm × 4 cm × 4 cm.

Two different setups are used: in particular, on 9 eggplants, the electrodes are placed with an inter-electrodic distance of 12 mm; on the remaining 20 eggplants, the inter-electrodic distance is 5 mm. Therefore, for the sake of clarity, the two different setups (12 and 5 mm) will be discussed separately.

- *12-mm setup:* Four FIAB PG500 gel electrodes are placed on the prepared eggplants. The electrodes of 14 mm × 36 mm are obtained by cutting lengthwise in half the full electrode of 28 mm × 36 mm. A preliminary impedance measurement is carried out for each sample, by imposing a sinusoidal voltage amplitude of 20 mV, at a frequency of 1 kHz. This measurement, performed before the infiltration, allows to improve inter-species reproducibility. Then, the total amount of insulin (0.25 ml) is administered 8 mm below the surface, by 5 consecutive steps of 0.05 ml. The insulin, Lilly's Humalog, of fast type, consists of a solution with 100 UI/ml, where each UI indicates 0.0347 mg of human insulin. The insulin is administered using a commercial pen and a dedicated needle (PIC Insumed 31 G syringe) with 31 G × 8 mm. G stands for Gauge, an internationally-used scale for sizing the thickness of a needle; in particular, the needle of 31 G has a diameter of 0.41 mm.

- *5-mm setup:* This setup provides different inter-electrode distance, injection depth, and amount of the injected insulin. The main purpose is to improve the instrument sensitivity, to emulate the actual condition of use, and to enhance as much as possible the benefit in diagnostic-therapeutic applications. Thus, two electrodes FIAB PG500 28 mm × 36 mm are cut lengthwise to obtain four electrodes of 7 mm × 36 mm. The fast insulin is injected by a 100 U/ml Insulin Pen at a 4 mm depth. A total amount of 10 IU dosage (i.e., 100 μl of solution) is injected in each single experiment, by five consecutive injections of 2 IU (i.e., 20 μl of insulin solution). The selected administered amount, as well as the used device, are close to the insulin injection technique and doses, commonly used in diabetes treatments.

For both setups, 5 mm and 12 mm, impedance measurements are repeated to reduce the uncertainty. The following subsections deal with the analysis of the main parameters useful for metrological characterization.

8.1.2 Drift

Drift refers to continuous or incremental change in indication over time, due to changes in the metrological properties of a measuring system or reference material [152]. In this context, drift arises from the evaporation of the water contained within the eggplant, which changes the impedance; as well as from the electrodes degradation, with the consequent electrolytic gel penetration into the eggplants. In particular, this latter has a significant impact on the impedance measurement [2].

The drift impact on the measured impedance is attenuated by the four-wires configuration. In Fig. 8.1, the trends of electrolyte gel penetration are illustrated for both the two-wires and the four-wires configuration. In the two-wires configuration, the progressive penetration of the electrolyte gel induces a decrease in contact impedance within 160 min. On the other hand, the four-wires configuration significantly reduces this effect, and the drift is reduced to 2.9 %.

8.1.3 Sensitivity

The sensitivity is defined as the ratio between the minimum variations in the response of a measuring system and the corresponding minimum appreciable variation in the measured quantity [152]. In this case, the Insulin Meter sensitivity is assessed as the slope of the linear model for the two different setups. For the 12-mm setup, the average values is equal to 24.7 ml^{-1}, meanwhile, for

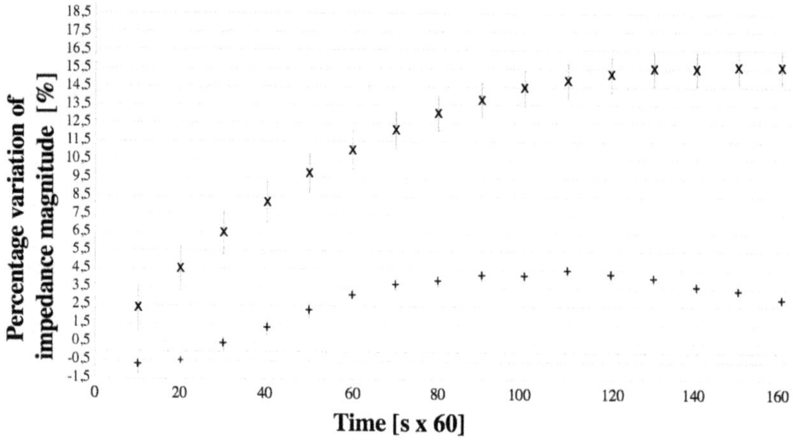

FIGURE 8.1
Dried eggplant drift (average on 10 measurements) in two-wires (×) and four-wires (+) configuration [8].

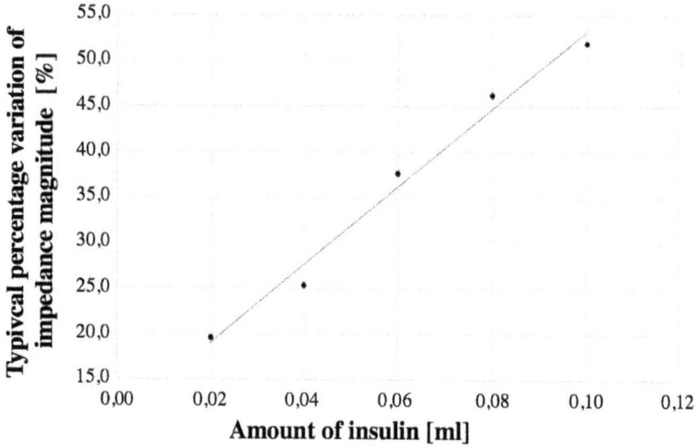

FIGURE 8.2
Percentage impedance magnitude variation vs amount of insulin solution in in-vitro experiments in 5-mm setup [8].

the 5-mm setup the average value is 497.3 ml^{-1}. Specifically, a variation of 1 ml of insulin generates a percentage impedance variation of 497.3 %, compared to the initial impedance measured before the injection.

The typical trend of the 5-mm setup on eggplants is shown in Fig. 8.2, in terms of the percentage change in impedance corresponding to the drug amount. Therefore, a sensitivity improvement of 20 % due to the 4-wire configuration is highlighted [2].

TABLE 8.1
Nonlinearity of the Insulin Meter for the 5-mm setup.

Eggplant sample	Generic %	Personalized %
# 1	9,7	4,6
# 2	5,3	5,1
# 3	4,6	4,6
# 4	5,2	1,6
# 5	9,9	9,8
# 6	1,6	1,6
# 7	3,2	1,4
# 8	4,8	3,4
# 9	6,8	4,4
# 10	6,1	5,1
# 11	3,7	2,0
# 12	3,9	2,2
# 13	4,5	3,9
# 14	5,0	4,8
# 15	2,5	2,5
# 16	4,6	3,3
# 17	2,8	2,5
# 18	11,5	9,9
# 19	4,8	2,3
# 20	9,5	6,0
Mean	5.5±0.6	4.0±0.5

8.1.4 Nonlinearity

By means of one-way ANOVA, the nonlinearity is determined as the standard deviation of the residuals of the linear model. For the 5-mm setup, the typical percentage values (expressed as the average ± 1-σ of the sample mean) are reported in Tab. 8.1, both for personalized and the generic model. In particular, the nonlinearity, exhibited by the personalized model, is always lower than the the generic model.

8.1.5 Repeatability

The repeatability condition of measurement represents a condition, out of a set of conditions that includes the same measurement procedure, same operators, same measuring system, same operating conditions and same location, and replicate measurements on the same or similar objects over a short period of time. A condition of measurement is a repeatability condition only with respect to a specified set of repeatability conditions [152].

For both the setups, 12 mm and 5 mm, the 1-σ repeatability is assessed as the percentage variation relative to the initial impedance value, at varying

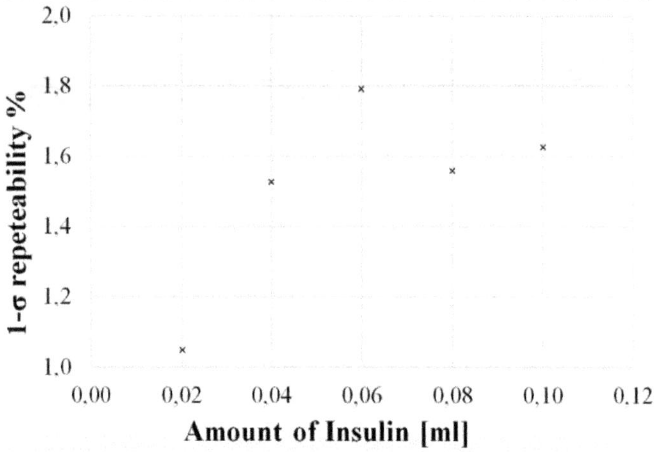

FIGURE 8.3
1-σ repeatability vs amount of injected drug in-vitro in the case of the 12 mm needle [8], as an example.

the amount of injected drug. The trends for both the setups is illustrated in Fig. 8.3. In particular, in the 12 mm setup, an average percentage values of 0.31 % is determined, meanwhile, a value of 1.3 % is achieved for the 5-mm setup.

8.1.6 Reproducibility

Generally, the reproducibility refers to the closeness of the agreement between measurements of the same quantity carried out in different conditions [152]. In this case, for the 12-mm setup, the 1-σ individual reproducibility of 0.1 % is assessed for the personalized model; while, for the generic model, the value is 0.7 %. Instead, the optimal setup presents a reproducibility of 2.4 % for the personalized solution and 2.7 % for the generic solution.

8.1.7 Accuracy

Accuracy is defined as the closeness of the agreement between the measurement result and the reference value of a measurand [152]. It is assessed as the RMS of the deterministic error. In Figs. 8.4, the accuracy is reported at varying the amount of injected insulin for both the 12-mm (A), and the 5-mm setup (B). In both the cases, the results of the personalized (+) and the generic model (×), respectively, are highlighted.

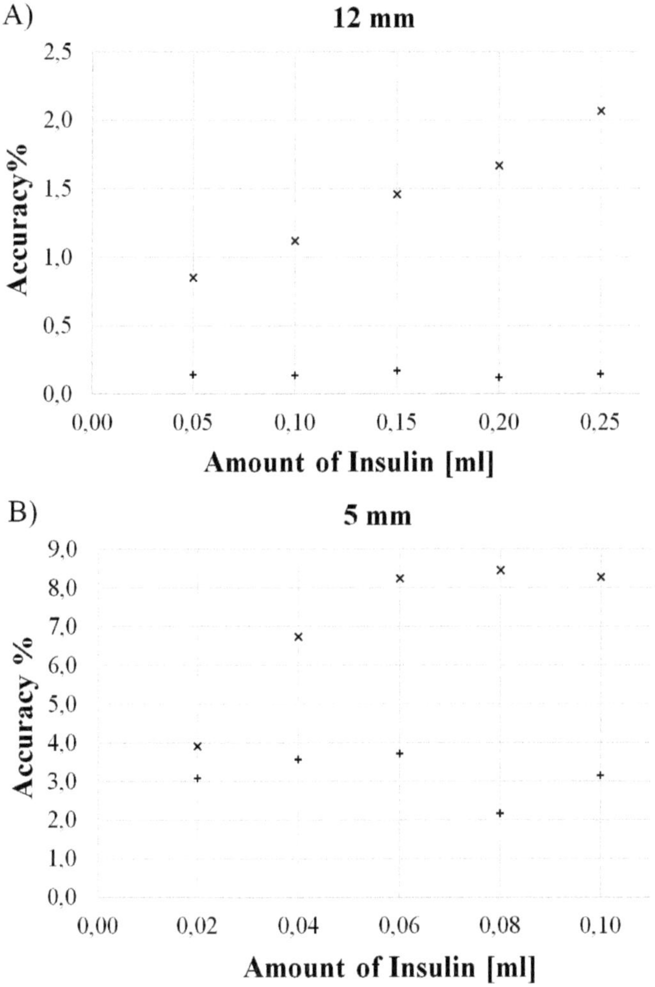

FIGURE 8.4
Percentage accuracy of the personalized (+) and the generic (×) model vs amount of insulin, in-vitro experiments for (A) the 12-mm and (B) the 5-mm setup [8].

8.2 Ex-vivo Metrological Characterization

As already highlighted in the previous chapters, the similarity between pig and human tissues is confirmed by several studies [160]. In particular, the membrane permeability, as well as the epidermal thickness and the lipid part, are indicated to be very similar to the human one [158,159]. Therefore, non-perfused abdominal muscles from several pigs are used to test the instrument, before to start the experiments on human volunteers.

Ex-vivo tests are carried out on 15 samples of pig tissues. Room temperature and relative humidity are 25 °C, and 50 %, respectively. All relevant guidelines and regulations are respected during the experiments. A local abattoir supplied the pig tissues samples, in compliance with the regulations on domestic animals intended for human consumption. No animals suffered or were killed as a result of the experiments.

Each pig muscle was cut to the dimensions of 7 cm × 7 cm × 4 cm. A total of 10 insulin units (IU) are injected at a depth of 4 mm via insulin pen. The insulin administration is articulated in five steps of 2 IU corresponding to 20 μl of insulin solution. The metrological characteristics are expressed analogously as for the eggplants experiment.

The typical relationship between the amount of insulin injected and the percentage variation of the impedance magnitude is reported in Fig. 8.5.

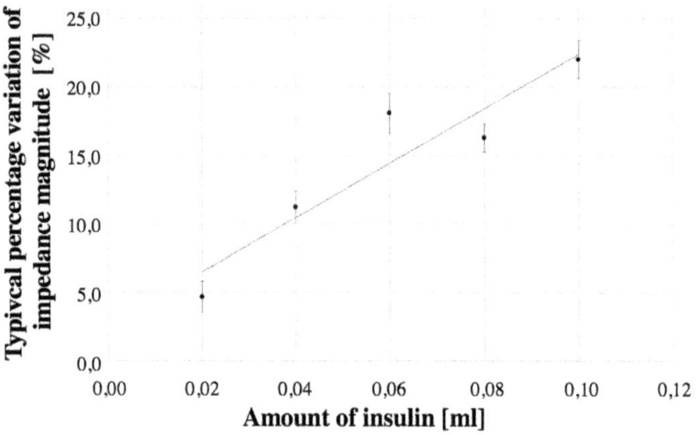

FIGURE 8.5
Typical percentage impedance magnitude variation vs insulin solution in ex-vivo experiments [8].

The sensitivity, the 1-σ repeatability, 1-σ repeatability the reproducibility, the nonlinearity, and the accuracy assessed both in the pig and in the eggplant tests are reported in Table 8.2, for the sake of the reader easiness. The same setup based on an electrode gap of 5 mm is considered for a more reliable results comparison. As reported in Figs. 8.4 (B) and 8.6, the personalized model performs better than the generic model, in terms of 1-σ repeatability and percentage accuracy.

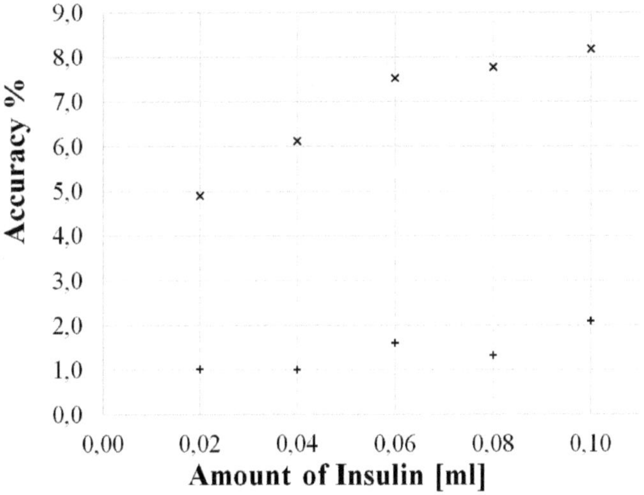

FIGURE 8.6
Percentage accuracy of personalized (+) and generic (×) model vs amount of drug in ex-vivo experiments [8].

TABLE 8.2
Metrological characteristics of pig abdominal non-perfused muscle and egg-plants.

	Pig	Dried Eggplant
Sensitivity [ml^{-1}]	157.2	497.3
nonlinearity [%]	2.1	4.0
1-σ repeatability [%]	1.6	1.3
Reproducibility [%]	2.4	1.9
Accuracy [%]	1.4	3.2

8.3 Preliminary in-vivo Test

The previously presented Insulin Meter is used for some in-vivo tests on a human subject affected by type-1 diabetes. The experimental campaign is approved by the Ethical Review Board of the University of Naples Federico II. The volunteer is a patient already undergoing diabetic therapy. The therapy includes bolus doses[1] of fast insulin administered in variable quantities 20

[1] A bolus dose is the insulin specifically assumed at meal times to keep blood glucose levels under control after food ingestion. Bolus insulin needs to act quickly and thus, short-acting insulin or rapid-acting insulin are required.

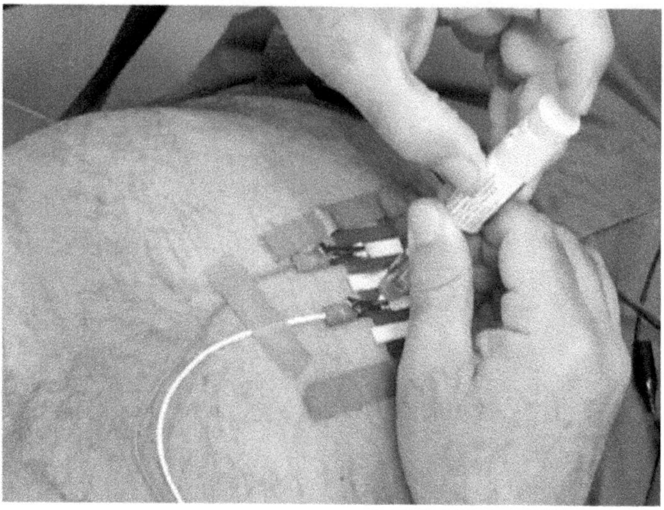

FIGURE 8.7
Insulin injection during in-vivo experiments [8].

min before meals. A regimen of basal-bolus injection involves carrying out a number of injections through the day, usually at each meal, in order to roughly attempt to emulate how a non-diabetic person's body provides insulin. In particular, Lilly's Humalog Insulin (100 U/ml), fast-acting insulin lispro injectable suspension, is used in a configuration of pre-filled commercial pen of 3 ml.

Impedance magnitude measurements are carried out on the patient by means of the Insulin Meter during the insulin bolus injection. The experimental setup is characterized by an injection depth of 4 mm and an inter-electrodes distance of 5 mm. The patient therapeutic value planned for the bolus is 0.10 ml and it is administered by successive steps of 0.02 ml (Fig. 8.7).

The impedance is measured after each injection step following the same protocol adopted in in-vitro and ex-vivo tests. The typical result of the experiment is reported in Fig. 8.8. Because of the variation of the amount of the injected insulin, there is a monotonous trend in the impedance variation compared to the initial value. The instrument sensitivity results compatible with the typical clinical insulin dosage. A linear model is suitable for describing the trend of the phenomenon for human subjects, already identified in the in-vitro and the ex-vivo tests. The Insulin Meter is upgraded after the first measurement session (Tab. 8.3, first row) with the purpose to improve the repeatability and did not allow to appreciate resolutions below 2 U. The following parameters are optimized: (i) applied voltage, increased up to the limits allowed by safety rules, and (ii) connection impedance exhibited by cables and contacts, respectively.

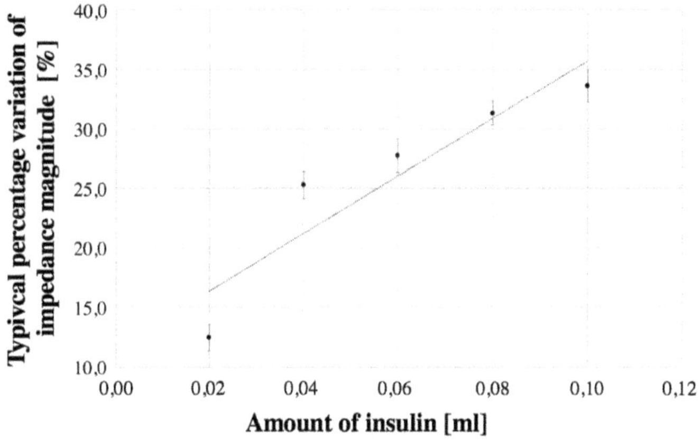

FIGURE 8.8
Typical percentage impedance magnitude variation vs insulin solution in the in-vivo experiments [8].

Subsequently, for further two months, the subject is involved in new tests, for a total of 300 measurements divided into daily sessions of 50 measurements. Compared to the first test session, the 1-σ repeatability is on average increased by an order of magnitude (Tab. 8.3, last column). The increase in repeatability allowed, among other advantages, to double the resolution of the steps of the measured quantity (from 2 IU to 1 IU per step).

The well-known problem of reproducibility for bioimpedance measurements [13] is confirmed by the experiments. In particular, poor reproducibility is experienced also at intra-individual level, mainly due to the skin moisture and skin barrier alterations [209]. The subject exhibits an average initial impedance value of 157 Ω calculated over six measurement sessions. The associated uncertainty is 42 Ω. The wide variability of the initial impedance value is not attributable to the different frequency of the stimulus signal. In fact, the variation between the sessions resulted significant even with the same applied frequency. Also the sensitivity exhibits low reproducibility at varying the measurement sessions: the uncertainty band is 80 ml^{-1}, almost equivalent to the average value of 98 ml^{-1}.

The described experiments proved to be effective in overcoming the impact of inter- and intra-individual nonreproducibility. The instrument allows the customization of the insulin appearance/disappearance model at each administration. Thus, the measurement non-repeatability is the only contribution to the uncertainty. The 1-σ repeatability is lower than 0.5 % after the optimization of the Insulin Meter. Even considering the worst-case sensitivity of 47 ml^{-1}, in case of a typical bolus dosage of 10 IU (e.g., 10 ml for concentration level of 100 IU/ml), a significant variation of 4.7 % of the initial impedance, or 10 times greater than the 1-σ repeatability, can be appreciated.

TABLE 8.3
In-vivo experimental results.

Dosage [IU * nr. step]	**Frequency** [kHz]	**Initial Impedance Value** [Ω]	**Sensitivity** [ml^{-1}]	**non linearity** [%]	**1-σ repeatability** [%]
2 IU * 5	1	343	242	16	4.17
	1	220	−113	12.1	0.72
	10	179	408	3.8	0.39
1 IU * 6	10	56	−101	6.5	0.41
	50	78	197	5.5	0.41
	50	66	−47	13.5	0.31

9

Orthopaedics

CONTENTS

In this chapter, the personalized model of the human knee is validated experimentally for enhancing the inter-individual reproducibility of a measurement method, presented in Chapter 6, for monitoring Non-Steroidal Anti-Inflammatory Drugs (NSAIDs) after transdermal delivery. The experimental validation includes two main steps: (*i*) identify the generic model, and (*ii*), after a sensitivity analysis aimed to reduce the computational burden, optimize the parameters to personalize the model. The optimization algorithm allows to find out the electrical parameters of each subject by experimental impedance spectroscopy data. The personalized model, based only on seven parameters, achieves a worst-case reconstruction error lower than 3 %. Finally, the personalized knee model and the optimization algorithm are validated in vivo by an experimental campaign on twenty volunteers with an average error of 2 %.

9.1 Experimental Validation of the Knee Generic Model

The generic knee FEM model, presented in Chapter 6, is validated by means of an experimental campaign. The average impedance values, collected during the tests on twenty subjects, are adopted as reference for the model validation.

DOI: 10.1201/9781003170143-9

9.1.1 Test Protocol and Setup

The experimental campaign enrolled 20 health young volunteers, 70 % women and 30 % men. Before collecting participants' data, the researchers clearly explain to the volunteers the scientific protocol, the purpose of the research, the benefits and the risks of the participation, and the kind of information to be collected, as well as the data deidentification and anonymization. Measurements are carried out according to the relevant guidelines and regulations. The experimental protocol, as a whole, was approved by the relevant ethics committee [11].

Once the informed consent, containing all the above mentioned information, are signed by the volunteers, their physiological parameters (sex, age, knee circumference, and body mass index BMI) are recorded. In particular, the average age of the volunteers is 24 ± 10 years, the knee circumference 38 cm ± 10 cm, and the BMI is 25 kg/m^2 ± 5 kg/m^2. The selected volunteers do not present any diseases, wounds, inflammation or underwent past knee surgery. Moreover, they are asked to avoid the use of moisturizers or oils the measurement day, in order to avoid problems with the electrodes application. The volunteers are asked to remove all the metallic objects and to sit comfortably on a chair completely isolated from the ground by means of a rubber mat. During the measurements, the volunteers are required to avoid movements and to touch metallic components. A battery-powered laptop gathers the data collected by the instrument. Effects of parasitic capacitances are minimized by making equipotential the patient and the instrument chassis, thanks to an electrocardiogram clamp electrode, positioned on the right ankle.

Subsequently, the measurements are carried out by the Analog Devices boards, previously described in Chapter 5. They are connected to the volunteers by means of four electrodes. The boards are included into a 15.0 cm × 17.0 cm × 4.5 cm plastic and aluminium casing; the device is never connected to the main supply, but powered by a USB cable connected to the laptop, in order to guarantee safety standards (Fig. 9.1). Moreover, in order to guarantee an adequate warm up, all the instruments are switched on at least one hour before starting the experiment. The four electrodes, placed around the knee, as shown in Fig. 9.2, are connected to the boards by means of four clips placed on a TPU (Thermoplastic Polyurethane) support. The customized support can adapt to different knee conformation and guarantees a stable measurement set up due to its durability and slightly malleability. The pre-gelled electrodes, (FIAB PG500) coated with a bio-compatible gel, are used to further the adherence of the electrodes to the skin surface. The impedance measurement are carried out by exploring thirteen frequency values in the frequency spectrum 1 Hz to 49 kHz. The laboratory temperature and humidity are monitored during all the experiments.

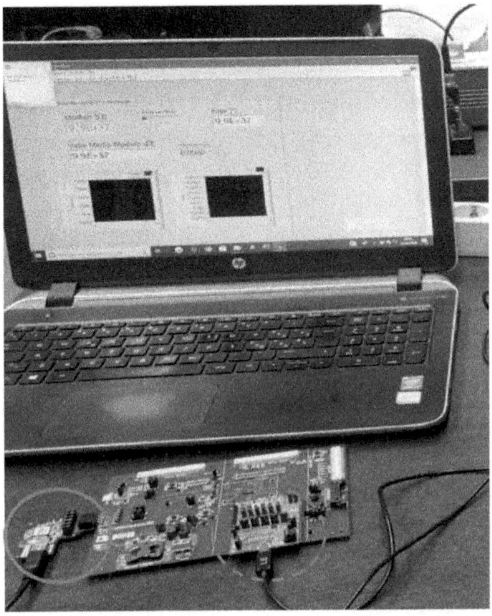

FIGURE 9.1
Experimental set up: The motherboard connected to a laptop PC by the USB-SW/UART-EMUZ (circled with solid line); and the daughterboard 4W-BIO3Z (circled with dashed line) connected to four electrodes on the knee by clip adapters.

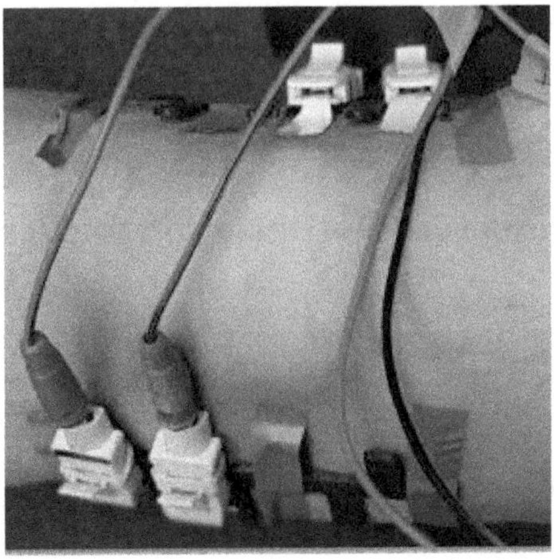

FIGURE 9.2
Four-wire electrodes applied to the knee opposite sides using a TPU support.

9.1.2 Preliminary Results

The impedance spectroscopy results are shown in Fig. 9.3 in terms of mean of impedance magnitude at each frequency and 1-σ reproducibility error bars on all the subjects. High values of standard deviation of a single data reveal a significant inter-individual variability. The percentage is computed with respect to the mean values (24 % at low frequencies and 16 % at high frequency). This point out the need for optimizing the knee parameters. However, the measured mean impedance values are compatible with the values generated by simulations of the generic model presented in Chapter 6.

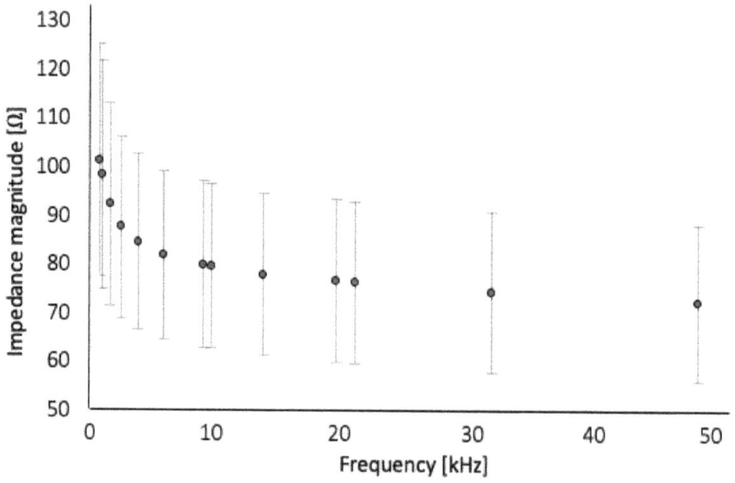

FIGURE 9.3
Impedance magnitude spectroscopy: mean (dots) 1-σ reproducibility (error bars) on all the 20 subjects.

9.2 Knee Parameters Optimization for Personalizing the Model

A parameter optimization enables the model to perform the task with acceptable inter-individual reproducibility. The parameters values reported in Tab. 6.3 are optimized to adapt them to the measured bioimpedance, in order to mitigate the effect of individual variability of the tissues and the approximation introduced by the model. Furthermore, the order of the operational space is also reduced by two steps: firstly, by extracting a parameters subset in a specific frequency range, secondly, by means of a sensitivity analysis. Thus, a suitable subset of the parameters appearing in the Cole-Cole equation is extracted according to the spectroscope frequency range. As matter of fact, some Cole-Cole parameters are fully operational only in a specific frequency range.

The knee-model electrical behaviour is personalized by adapting the reference values shown in Tab. 9.1 for fitting individual experimental data. However, considering their large number (eighty in all), the parameters have to be reduced. To this aim, the parameters most affecting the bioimpedance magnitude spectrum are determined by a sensitivity analysis.

9.2.1 Sensitivity Analysis

Before the sensitivity analysis, the number of the parameters is reduced, for each tissue, by assessing the frequency range, and by considering the effects of each relaxation on the spectrum of the actual dielectric permittivity.

The sensitivity analysis evaluates how the model parameters influence the output or design requirements. It allows to identify the parameters to be measured accurately and to be determined for patient-specific applications.

In particular, the parameters to be analyzed are referred to the equation 6.1 of the effective dielectric permittivity. Then, a one-at-a-time-parameter sensitivity analysis is carried out in order to determine the parameters most affecting the bioimpedance magnitude spectrum. The resulting seven Cole-Cole parameters most impacting on simulated bioimpedance magnitude are reported in Tab. 9.1.

A Nelder-Mead simplex optimization procedure [210] is carried out. The actual values of the seven parameters extracted by the sensitivity analysis in step 1, are identified, in order to fit the individual bioimpedance magnitude spectrum within a tolerance lower than 5 %. Therefore, the prediction error is assessed in terms of relative difference between reconstructed and experimental bioimpedance magnitude:

$$\varepsilon_{fit} = \frac{||Z_{exp}(\omega_k) - Z_{sim}(\omega_k)||}{||Z_{exp}(\omega_k)||} \tag{9.1}$$

where Z_{exp} is the impedance value measured experimentally, Z_{sim} the impedance value simulated by the model, and ω_k the experimental angular frequency.

This definition is used to identify the men/women with values of bioimpedance magnitude spectrum farthest from the male/female average. Later, these subjects are exploited to validate the knee joint model in terms of individual fitting. Four out of the twenty volunteers are chosen for validation, two per sex: namely, with the highest and the lowest average bioimpedance magnitude between the males and the females. They are labelled as MH and ML, respectively, for the males, and FH and FL, respectively, for the females. The optimization returns the individual impedance spectroscopy curve fitting, within a reconstruction error in 1 % to 3 %. Figs. 9.4 and 9.5 show the results in terms of bioimpedance magnitude fitting for male and female subjects, respectively.

The parameters subjected to the optimization are reported in Tab. 9.1. The values obtaining by the optimization are reported in Tab. 9.2.

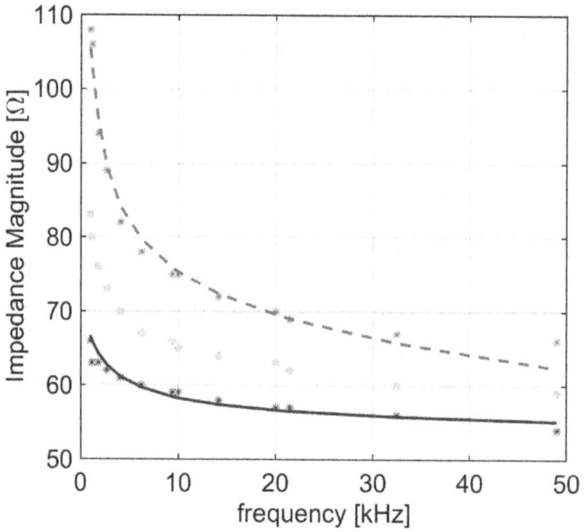

FIGURE 9.4
Impedance magnitude identification of male subjects: average impedance (green dotted line), experimental impedance (starred lines), fitted impedance (solid line), and fitted impedance (dashed line).

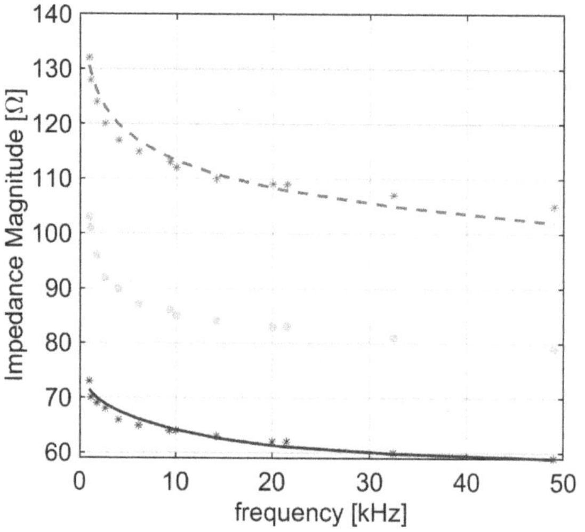

FIGURE 9.5
Impedance magnitude identification of female subjects: average impedance (green dotted line), experimental impedance (starred lines), fitted impedance (solid line), and fitted impedance (dashed line).

TABLE 9.1
The seven parameters used for personal model personalization.

	ε_∞	$\Delta\varepsilon_1$	τ_1	α_1	$\Delta\varepsilon_2$	τ_2	α_2	$\Delta\varepsilon_3$	τ_3	α_3	$\Delta\varepsilon_4$	τ_4	α_4	σ_{dc}
Dry Skin														
Wet Skin								×			×			
Fat													×	×
Muscle (Transverse)														
Muscle (Parallel)										×		×		×
Bone														

TABLE 9.2
Optimized value of Cole-Cole parameters for identified individuals outliers.

		Male		Female	
		M_L	M_H	F_L	F_H
Wet Skin	$\Delta\varepsilon_3$	5000	4412	5085	30612
	$\Delta\varepsilon_4$	75000	600	5000	30000
Fat	α_4	0.200	0.405	0.240	0.038
	σ_{dc} [S/m]	0.052	0.012	0.0321	0.034
Muscle (Parallel)	α_3	0.320	0.260	0.313	0.536
	τ_4 [ms]	5.896	4.142	5.421	3.184
	σ_{dc} [S/m]	0.224	0.068	0.015	0.074

9.3 Discussion

A personalized FEM model of knee for improving reproducibility in NSAIDs transdermal delivery measurement is described. The model geometry is based on five layers: bone, muscle, fat, wet skin and dry skin. Each layer thicknesses of layers is personalized according to sex, BMI index, and circumference of knee. Electrical characterization of the tissues takes into account their non ideal loss and dispersive behaviour by means of Cole-Cole model. The muscle tissue is characterized not only transversally: the parameters of the Cole-Cole equation of the parallel component are derived from experimental data available in the literature.

Personalized models are identified by tuning seven electrical parameters: less than 10 % of the initial amount. Models are validated on the subjects (two per sex) with extreme characteristics in an experimental campaign involving twenty volunteers. The results of the optimization proved the feasibility of personalizing the generic knee model to the specific characteristics of an individual. The error is assessed on the worst-case subjects with parameters farthest from the average trend. Seven parameters are sufficient to keep the maximum error below 3 %. Three parameters, belonged to the parallel component of the muscle layers, are identified through this study.

The personalization of a simplified knee FEM model with a low computational burden is proven to be feasible.

A forthcoming modelling of NSAIDs electrical behaviour in human tissues, combined with the personalized models, will allow a high-reproducible assessment of drug amount transdermally delivered.

Bibliography

[1] "Gr 1689rlc digibridge generalradio." Accessed: 2021-07-15.

[2] P. Arpaia, U. Cesaro, and N. Moccaldi, "Noninvasive measurement of transdermal drug delivery by impedance spectroscopy," *Scientific Reports*, vol. 7, p. 44647, 2017.

[3] G. Taguchi and M. S. Phadke, "Quality engineering through design optimization," in *Quality control, robust design, and the Taguchi method*, pp. 77–96, Springer, 1989.

[4] P. Arpaia, U. Cesaro, and N. Moccaldi, "A bioimpedance meter to measure drug in transdermal delivery," *IEEE Transactions on Instrumentation and Measurement*, vol. 67, no. 10, pp. 2324–2331, 2018.

[5] "Analog devices aducm350." Acessed: 2021-07-21.

[6] S. Kalra, A. Mithal, R. Sahay, M. John, A. Unnikrishnan, B. Saboo, S. Ghosh, D. Sanyal, L. J. Hirsch, V. Gupta, *et al.*, "Indian injection technique study: injecting complications, education, and the health care professional," *Diabetes Therapy*, vol. 8, no. 3, pp. 659–672, 2017.

[7] P. Arpaia, O. Cuomo, N. Moccaldi, A. Smarra, and M. Taglialatela, "Non-invasive real-time in-vivo monitoring of insulin absorption from subcutaneous tissues," in *Journal of Physics: Conference Series*, vol. 1065, p. 132008, IOP Publishing, 2018.

[8] P. Arpaia, U. Cesaro, M. Frosolone, N. Moccaldi, and M. Taglialatela, "A micro-bioimpedance meter for monitoring insulin bioavailability in personalized diabetes therapy," *Scientific Reports*, vol. 10, no. 1, pp. 1–11, 2020.

[9] P. Arpaia, U. Cesaro, P. Cimmino, and N. Moccaldi, "Drug under skin meter (dusm): a portable bio-impedance spectroscope for assessing transdermal drug delivery," in *The 14th IMEKO TC10 Workshop on Technical Diagnostics. Milano, Italy, June 26–28*, 2016.

[10] Doctorlib, "Atlas of anatomy 25 knee & leg," 2015–2019. [Online; accessed 21-July-2021].

[11] P. Arpaia, F. Crauso, S. Grassini, S. Minucci, N. Moccaldi, and I. Sannino, "Preliminary experimental identification of a fem human knee model," in *2020 IEEE International Symposium on Medical Measurements and Applications (MeMeA)*, pp. 1–6, IEEE, 2020.

[12] F. G. Jonathan Elsner, Sigal Portnoy, "Mri-based characterization of bone anatomy in the human knee for size matching of a medial meniscal implant," *Journal of Biomechanical Engineering*, vol. 132, no. 10, p. 101008, 2010.

[13] S. Gabriel, R. Lau, and C. Gabriel, "The dielectric properties of biological tissues: Ii. measurements in the frequency range 10 hz to 20 ghz," *Physics in Medicine & Biology*, vol. 41, no. 11, p. 2251, 1996.

[14] R. G. Trohman and J. E. Parrillo, "Direct current cardioversion: indications, techniques, and recent advances," *Critical Care Medicine*, vol. 28, no. 10, pp. N170–N173, 2000.

[15] T. S. Alster and J. R. Lupton, "Nonablative cutaneous remodeling using radiofrequency devices," *Clinics in Dermatology*, vol. 25, no. 5, pp. 487–491, 2007.

[16] M. Elman, I. Vider, Y. Harth, V. Gottfried, and A. Shemer, "Noninvasive therapy of wrinkles and lax skin using a novel multisource phase-controlled radio frequency system," *Journal of Cosmetic and Laser Therapy*, vol. 12, no. 2, pp. 81–86, 2010.

[17] S. Schwingenschuh, H. Scharfetter, Ø. G. Martinsen, B. Boulgaropoulos, T. Augustin, K. I. Tiffner, C. Dragatin, R. Raml, C. Hoefferer, E.-C. Prandl, *et al.*, "Assessment of skin permeability to topically applied drugs by skin impedance and admittance," *Physiological Measurement*, vol. 38, no. 11, p. N138, 2017.

[18] N. S. Sadick and Y. Makino, "Selective electro-thermolysis in aesthetic medicine: A review," *Lasers in Surgery and Medicine*, vol. 34, no. 2, pp. 91–97, 2004.

[19] Y. Harth and D. Lischinsky, "A novel method for real-time skin impedance measurement during radiofrequency skin tightening treatments," *Journal of Cosmetic Dermatology*, vol. 10, no. 1, pp. 24–29, 2011.

[20] E. B. Lack, J. D. Rachel, L. D'Andrea, and J. Corres, "Relationship of energy settings and impedance in different anatomic areas using a radiofrequency device," *Dermatologic Surgery*, vol. 31, no. 12, pp. 1668–1670, 2005.

[21] M. N. Padamwar, A. P. Pawar, A. V. Daithankar, and K. Mahadik, "Silk sericin as a moisturizer: an in vivo study," *Journal of Cosmetic Dermatology*, vol. 4, no. 4, pp. 250–257, 2005.

[22] I. H. Blank, "Factors which influence the water content of the stratum corneum," *Journal of Investigative Dermatology*, vol. 18, no. 6, pp. 433–440, 1952.

[23] S. Verdier-Sévrain and F. Bonté, "Skin hydration: a review on its molecular mechanisms," *Journal of Cosmetic Dermatology*, vol. 6, no. 2, pp. 75–82, 2007.

[24] X. Huang, W.-H. Yeo, Y. Liu, and J. A. Rogers, "Epidermal differential impedance sensor for conformal skin hydration monitoring," *Biointerphases*, vol. 7, no. 1, p. 52, 2012.

[25] L.-C. Gerhardt, V. Strässle, A. Lenz, N. D. Spencer, and S. Derler, "Influence of epidermal hydration on the friction of human skin against textiles," *Journal of the Royal Society Interface*, vol. 5, no. 28, pp. 1317–1328, 2008.

[26] C. Blichmann and J. Serup, "Hydration studies on scaly hand eczema," *Contact Dermatitis*, vol. 16, no. 3, pp. 155–159, 1987.

[27] U. H. Birgersson, E. Birgersson, and S. Ollmar, "Estimating electrical properties and the thickness of skin with electrical impedance spectroscopy: Mathematical analysis and measurements," *Journal of Electrical Bioimpedance*, vol. 3, no. 1, pp. 51–60, 2012.

[28] K. Kontturi, L. Murtomäki, J. Hirvonen, P. Paronen, and A. Urtti, "Electrochemical characterization of human skin by impedance spectroscopy: the effect of penetration enhancers," *Pharmaceutical Research*, vol. 10, no. 3, pp. 381–385, 1993.

[29] L. Ventrelli, L. Marsilio Strambini, and G. Barillaro, "Microneedles for transdermal biosensing: current picture and future direction," *Advanced Healthcare Materials*, vol. 4, no. 17, pp. 2606–2640, 2015.

[30] O. G. Jepps, Y. Dancik, Y. G. Anissimov, and M. S. Roberts, "Modeling the human skin barrier—towards a better understanding of dermal absorption," *Advanced Drug Delivery Reviews*, vol. 65, no. 2, pp. 152–168, 2013.

[31] S. Huclova, D. Baumann, M. S. Talary, and J. Fröhlich, "Sensitivity and specificity analysis of fringing-field dielectric spectroscopy applied to a multi-layer system modelling the human skin," *Physics in Medicine & Biology*, vol. 56, no. 24, p. 7777, 2011.

[32] J. Phipps, R. Padmanabhan, and G. Lattin, "Transport of ionic species through skin," *Solid State Ionics*, vol. 28, pp. 1778–1783, 1988.

[33] J. E. Riviere and M. C. Heit, "Electrically-assisted transdermal drug delivery," *Pharmaceutical Research*, vol. 14, no. 6, pp. 687–697, 1997.

[34] T. Yamamoto and Y. Yamamoto, "Electrical properties of the epidermal stratum corneum," *Medical and Biological Engineering*, vol. 14, no. 2, pp. 151–158, 1976.

[35] N. H. Yoshida and M. S. Roberts, "Solute molecular size and transdermal iontophoresis across excised human skin," *Journal of Controlled Release*, vol. 25, no. 3, pp. 177–195, 1993.

[36] V. Aguilella, M. Belaya, and V. Levadny, "Passive transport of small ions through human stratum corneum," *Journal of Controlled Release*, vol. 44, no. 1, pp. 11–18, 1997.

[37] A. K. Banga and Y. W. Chien, "Iontophoretic delivery of drugs: fundamentals, developments and biomedical applications," *Journal of Controlled Release*, vol. 7, no. 1, pp. 1–24, 1988.

[38] J. J. Ackmann and M. A. Seitz, "Methods of complex impedance measurements in biologic tissue.," *Critical Reviews in Biomedical Engineering*, vol. 11, no. 4, pp. 281–311, 1984.

[39] L. E. Sebar, L. Iannucci, E. Angelini, S. Grassini, and M. Parvis, "Electrochemical impedance spectroscopy system based on a teensy board," *IEEE Transactions on Instrumentation and Measurement*, vol. 70, pp. 1–9, 2020.

[40] P. Arpaia, F. Clemente, C. Romanucci, and A. Zanesco, "Experimental characterization of an eis-based method for low-invasive diagnosis of prosthesis osseointegration," in *XVIII IMEKO Word Congress, Rio de Janeiro (Brasil)*, pp. 17–22, 2006.

[41] S. Naito, M. Hoshi, and S. Yagihara, "Microwave dielectric analysis of human stratum corneum in vivo," *Biochimica et Biophysica Acta (BBA)-General Subjects*, vol. 1381, no. 3, pp. 293–304, 1998.

[42] S. Grimnes and O. G. Martinsen, "Cole electrical impedance model-a critique and an alternative," *IEEE Transactions on Biomedical Engineering*, vol. 52, no. 1, pp. 132–135, 2004.

[43] U. Birgersson, E. Birgersson, P. Åberg, I. Nicander, and S. Ollmar, "Non-invasive bioimpedance of intact skin: mathematical modeling and experiments," *Physiological Measurement*, vol. 32, no. 1, p. 1, 2011.

[44] Z. Erdogan Iyigun, D. Selamoglu, G. Alco, K. N. Pilancı, C. Ordu, F. Agacayak, F. Elbüken, A. Bozdogan, S. Ilgun, F. Guler Uysal, *et al.*, "Bioelectrical impedance for detecting and monitoring lymphedema in patients with breast cancer. preliminary results of the florence nightingale breast study group," *Lymphatic Research and Biology*, vol. 13, no. 1, pp. 40–45, 2015.

[45] P. Åberg, U. Birgersson, P. Elsner, P. Mohr, and S. Ollmar, "Electrical impedance spectroscopy and the diagnostic accuracy for malignant melanoma," *Experimental Dermatology*, vol. 20, no. 8, pp. 648–652, 2011.

[46] U. G. Kyle, I. Bosaeus, A. D. De Lorenzo, P. Deurenberg, M. Elia, J. M. Gómez, B. L. Heitmann, L. Kent-Smith, J.-C. Melchior, M. Pirlich, *et al.*, "Bioelectrical impedance analysis—part i: review of principles and methods," *Clinical Nutrition*, vol. 23, no. 5, pp. 1226–1243, 2004.

[47] C. Earthman, D. Traughber, J. Dobratz, and W. Howell, "Bioimpedance spectroscopy for clinical assessment of fluid distribution and body cell mass," *Nutrition in Clinical Practice*, vol. 22, no. 4, pp. 389–405, 2007.

[48] T. G. Lohman and S. B. Going, "Body composition assessment for development of an international growth standard for preadolescent and adolescent children," *Food and Nutrition Bulletin*, vol. 27, no. 4_suppl5, pp. S314–S325, 2006.

[49] K. R. Foster and H. C. Lukaski, "Whole-body impedance–what does it measure?," *The American Journal of Clinical Nutrition*, vol. 64, no. 3, pp. 388S–396S, 1996.

[50] R. Gudivaka, D. Schoeller, R. Kushner, and M. Bolt, "Single-and multifrequency models for bioelectrical impedance analysis of body water compartments," *Journal of Applied Physiology*, vol. 87, no. 3, pp. 1087–1096, 1999.

[51] J. Matthie, B. Zarowitz, A. De Lorenzo, A. Andreoli, K. Katzarski, G. Pan, and P. Withers, "Analytic assessment of the various bioimpedance methods used to estimate body water," *Journal of Applied Physiology*, vol. 84, no. 5, pp. 1801–1816, 1998.

[52] R. C. Janaway, S. L. Percival, and A. S. Wilson, "Decomposition of human remains," in *Microbiology and Aging*, pp. 313–334, Springer, 2009.

[53] T. Lohman, Z. Wang, and S. B. Going, *Human Body Composition*, vol. 918. Human Kinetics, 2005.

[54] C. Gagnon, J. Ménard, A. Bourbonnais, J.-L. Ardilouze, J.-P. Baillargeon, A. C. Carpentier, and M.-F. Langlois, "Comparison of foot-to-foot and hand-to-foot bioelectrical impedance methods in a population with a wide range of body mass indices," *Metabolic Syndrome and Related Disorders*, vol. 8, no. 5, pp. 437–441, 2010.

[55] R. V. Patel, E. L. Peterson, N. Silverman, and B. J. Zarowitz, "Estimation of total body and extracellular water in post-coronary artery bypass graft surgical patients using single and multiple frequency bioimpedance," *Critical Care Medicine*, vol. 24, no. 11, pp. 1824–1828, 1996.

[56] M. G. O. Rikkert, P. Deurenberg, R. W. Jansen, M. A. van't Hof, and W. H. Hoefnagels, "Validation of multi-frequency bioelectrical impedance analysis in detecting changes in fluid balance of geriatric patients," *Journal of the American Geriatrics Society*, vol. 45, no. 11, pp. 1345–1351, 1997.

[57] R. Kushner, D. A. Schoeller, C. R. Fjeld, and L. Danford, "Is the impedance index (ht2/r) significant in predicting total body water?," *The American Journal of Clinical Nutrition*, vol. 56, no. 5, pp. 835–839, 1992.

[58] T. K. Bera, "Bioelectrical impedance methods for noninvasive health monitoring: a review," *Journal of Medical Engineering*, vol. 2014, 2014.

[59] R. F. Kushner, R. Gudivaka, and D. A. Schoeller, "Clinical characteristics influencing bioelectrical impedance analysis measurements," *The American Journal of Clinical Nutrition*, vol. 64, no. 3, pp. 423S–427S, 1996.

[60] L. Garby, O. Lammert, and E. Nielsen, "Negligible effects of previous moderate physical activity and changes in environmental temperature on whole body electrical impedance.," *European Journal of Clinical Nutrition*, vol. 44, no. 7, pp. 545–546, 1990.

[61] M. Marra, R. Sammarco, A. De Lorenzo, F. Iellamo, M. Siervo, A. Pietrobelli, L. M. Donini, L. Santarpia, M. Cataldi, F. Pasanisi, *et al.*, "Assessment of body composition in health and disease using bioelectrical impedance analysis (bia) and dual energy x-ray absorptiometry (dxa): a critical overview," *Contrast Media & Molecular imaging*, vol. 2019, 2019.

[62] N. C. Battistini and G. Bedogni, "Impedenza bioelettrica e composizione corporea," Edra, 1998.

[63] N. I. Tanaka, M. Miyatani, Y. Masuo, T. Fukunaga, and H. Kanehisa, "Applicability of a segmental bioelectrical impedance analysis for predicting the whole body skeletal muscle volume," *Journal of Applied Physiology*, vol. 103, no. 5, pp. 1688–1695, 2007.

[64] B. Thomas, B. Cornish, L. Ward, and M. Patterson, "A comparison of segmental and wrist-to-ankle methodologies of bioimpedance analysis," *Applied Radiation and Isotopes*, vol. 49, no. 5-6, pp. 477–478, 1998.

[65] R. Aaron and C. Shiffman, "Using localized impedance measurements to study muscle changes in injury and disease," *Annals of the New York Academy of Sciences*, vol. 904, no. 1, pp. 171–180, 2000.

[66] M. Marra, B. Da Prat, C. Montagnese, A. Caldara, R. Sammarco, F. Pasanisi, and R. Corsetti, "Segmental bioimpedance analysis in professional cyclists during a three week stage race," *Physiological Measurement*, vol. 37, no. 7, p. 1035, 2016.

[67] M. Marra, A. Caldara, C. Montagnese, E. De Filippo, F. Pasanisi, F. Contaldo, and L. Scalfi, "Bioelectrical impedance phase angle in constitutionally lean females, ballet dancers and patients with anorexia nervosa," *European Journal of Clinical Nutrition*, vol. 63, no. 7, pp. 905–908, 2009.

[68] L. Nescolarde, A. Piccoli, A. Román, A. Nunez, R. Morales, J. Tamayo, T. Doñate, and J. Rosell, "Bioelectrical impedance vector analysis in haemodialysis patients: relation between oedema and mortality," *Physiological Measurement*, vol. 25, no. 5, p. 1271, 2004.

[69] A. Piccoli, I. C.-B. S. Group, *et al.*, "Bioelectric impedance vector distribution in peritoneal dialysis patients with different hydration status," *Kidney International*, vol. 65, no. 3, pp. 1050–1063, 2004.

[70] F. W. Guglielmi, T. Mastronuzzi, L. Pietrini, A. Panarese, C. Panella, and A. Francavilla, "The rxc graph in evaluating and monitoring fluid balance in patients with liver cirrhosis," *Annals of the New York Academy of Sciences*, vol. 873, no. 1, pp. 105–111, 1999.

[71] S.-H. Liu, D.-C. Cheng, and C.-H. Su, "A cuffless blood pressure measurement based on the impedance plethysmography technique," *Sensors*, vol. 17, no. 5, p. 1176, 2017.

[72] A. Brahme, *Comprehensive biomedical physics.* Newnes, 2014.

[73] G. Jindal, S. Pedhnekar, S. Nerurkar, K. Masand, D. Gupta, H. Deshmukh, J. Bapu, and G. Parulkar, "Diagnosis of venous disorders using impedance plethysmography.," *Journal of Postgraduate Medicine*, vol. 36, no. 3, p. 158, 1990.

[74] S. Kerai *et al.*, "The impedance cardiography technique in medical diagnosis," *Medical Technologies Journal*, vol. 2, no. 3, pp. 232–244, 2018.

[75] N. Kuzmina, T. Talme, J. Lapins, and L. Emtestam, "Non-invasive preoperative assessment of basal cell carcinoma of nodular and superficial types," *Skin Research and Technology*, vol. 11, no. 3, pp. 196–200, 2005.

[76] D. Atlas *et al.*, "International diabetes federation," *IDF Diabetes Atlas, 7th edn. Brussels, Belgium: International Diabetes Federation*, 2015.

[77] C. Chen, X.-L. Zhao, Z.-H. Li, Z.-G. Zhu, S.-H. Qian, and A. J. Flewitt, "Current and emerging technology for continuous glucose monitoring," *Sensors*, vol. 17, no. 1, p. 182, 2017.

[78] P. B. Luppa, C. Müller, A. Schlichtiger, and H. Schlebusch, "Point-of-care testing (poct): Current techniques and future perspectives," *TrAC Trends in Analytical Chemistry*, vol. 30, no. 6, pp. 887–898, 2011.

[79] A. K. Amerov, J. Chen, G. W. Small, and M. A. Arnold, "Scattering and absorption effects in the determination of glucose in whole blood by near-infrared spectroscopy," *Analytical Chemistry*, vol. 77, no. 14, pp. 4587–4594, 2005.

[80] S. N. Thennadil, J. L. Rennert, B. J. Wenzel, K. H. Hazen, T. L. Ruchti, and M. B. Block, "Comparison of glucose concentration in interstitial fluid, and capillary and venous blood during rapid changes in blood glucose levels," *Diabetes Technology & Therapeutics*, vol. 3, no. 3, pp. 357–365, 2001.

[81] S. K. Vashist, "Non-invasive glucose monitoring technology in diabetes management: A review," *Analytica Chimica Acta*, vol. 750, pp. 16–27, 2012.

[82] H. Heise and R. Marbach, "Human oral mucosa studies with varying blood glucose concentration by non-invasive atr-ft-ir-spectroscopy," *Cellular and Molecular Biology (Noisy-le-Grand, France)*, vol. 44, no. 6, pp. 899–912, 1998.

[83] B. P. Kovatchev, L. A. Gonder-Frederick, D. J. Cox, and W. L. Clarke, "Evaluating the accuracy of continuous glucose-monitoring sensors: continuous glucose–error grid analysis illustrated by therasense freestyle navigator data," *Diabetes Care*, vol. 27, no. 8, pp. 1922–1928, 2004.

[84] D. Li, Z. Pu, W. Liang, T. Liu, R. Wang, H. Yu, and K. Xu, "Non-invasive measurement of normal skin impedance for determining the volume of the transdermally extracted interstitial fluid," *Measurement*, vol. 62, pp. 215–221, 2015.

[85] J. Juansah and W. Yulianti, "Studies on electrical behavior of glucose using impedance spectroscopy," in *IOP Conference Series: Earth and Environmental Science*, vol. 31, p. 012039, IOP Publishing, 2016.

[86] J. Li, T. Igbe, Y. Liu, Z. Nie, W. Qin, L. Wang, and Y. Hao, "An approach for noninvasive blood glucose monitoring based on bioimpedance difference considering blood volume pulsation," *IEEE Access*, vol. 6, pp. 51119–51129, 2018.

[87] H. N. Mayrovitz, A. McClymont, and N. Pandya, "Skin tissue water assessed via tissue dielectric constant measurements in persons with and without diabetes mellitus," *Diabetes Technology & Therapeutics*, vol. 15, no. 1, pp. 60–65, 2013.

[88] H. N. Mayrovitz, I. Volosko, B. Sarkar, and N. Pandya, "Arm, leg, and foot skin water in persons with diabetes mellitus (dm) in relation to hba1c assessed by tissue dielectric constant (tdc) technology measured at 300 mhz," *Journal of Diabetes Science and Technology*, vol. 11, no. 3, pp. 584–589, 2017.

[89] R. Pradhan, A. Mitra, and S. Das, "Quantitative evaluation of blood glucose concentration using impedance sensing devices," *Journal of Electrical Bioimpedance*, vol. 4, no. 1, pp. 73–77, 2013.

[90] A. A. Farooqui, *Insulin Resistance as a Risk Factor in Visceral and Neurological Disorders.* Academic Press, 2020.

[91] P. Cryer, *Hypoglycemia in diabetes: pathophysiology, prevalence, and prevention.* American Diabetes Association, 2016.

[92] F. Zaccardi, D. Webb, Z. Htike, D. Youssef, K. Khunti, and M. Davies, "Efficacy and safety of sodium-glucose co-transporter-2 inhibitors in type 2 diabetes mellitus: systematic review and network meta-analysis," *Diabetes, Obesity and Metabolism*, vol. 18, no. 8, pp. 783–794, 2016.

[93] E. Carson and C. Cobelli, *Modelling methodology for physiology and medicine.* Newnes, 2013.

[94] J. G. Chase, G. M. Shaw, X.-W. Wong, T. Lotz, J. Lin, and C. E. Hann, "Model-based glycaemic control in critical care—a review of the state of the possible," *Biomedical Signal Processing and Control*, vol. 1, no. 1, pp. 3–21, 2006.

[95] R. N. Bergman, D. T. Finegood, and M. Ader, "Assessment of insulin sensitivity in vivo," *Endocrine Reviews*, vol. 6, no. 1, pp. 45–86, 1985.

[96] S. Salinari, A. Bertuzzi, and G. Mingrone, "Intestinal transit of a glucose bolus and incretin kinetics: a mathematical model with application to the oral glucose tolerance test," *American Journal of Physiology-Endocrinology and Metabolism*, vol. 300, no. 6, pp. E955–E965, 2011.

[97] E. J. Mansell, P. D. Docherty, and J. G. Chase, "Shedding light on grey noise in diabetes modelling," *Biomedical Signal Processing and Control*, vol. 31, pp. 16–30, 2017.

[98] E. Bekiari, K. Kitsios, H. Thabit, M. Tauschmann, E. Athanasiadou, T. Karagiannis, A.-B. Haidich, R. Hovorka, and A. Tsapas, "Artificial pancreas treatment for outpatients with type 1 diabetes: systematic review and meta-analysis," *bmj*, vol. 361, 2018.

[99] A. Caduff, E. Hirt, Y. Feldman, Z. Ali, and L. Heinemann, "First human experiments with a novel non-invasive, non-optical continuous glucose monitoring system," *Biosensors and Bioelectronics*, vol. 19, no. 3, pp. 209–217, 2003.

[100] S. A. Weinzimer, "Analysis: Pendra: the once and future noninvasive continuous glucose monitoring device?," *Diabetes Technology & Therapeutics*, vol. 6, no. 4, pp. 442–444, 2004.

[101] G. Dorsaf, M. Yacine, N. Khaled, *et al.*, "Non-invasive glucose monitoring: application and technologies," *Curr Trends Biomed Eng Biosci*, vol. 14, no. 1, p. 555878, 2018.

[102] K. R. Pitzer, S. Desai, T. Dunn, S. E. Jayalakshmi, J. Kennedy, J. A. Tamada, and R. O. Potts, "Detection of hypoglycemia with the glucowatch biographer," *Clinical Diabetology*, vol. 2, no. 4, pp. 307–314, 2001.

[103] M. Tierney, J. Tamada, R. Potts, L. Jovanovic, S. Garg, C. R. Team, *et al.*, "Clinical evaluation of the glucowatch® biographer: a continual, non-invasive glucose monitor for patients with diabetes," *Biosensors and Bioelectronics*, vol. 16, no. 9-12, pp. 621–629, 2001.

[104] R. Thibault, E. Le Gallic, M. Picard-Kossovsky, D. Darmaun, and A. Chambellan, "Assessment of nutritional status and body composition in patients with copd: comparison of several methods," *Revue des Maladies Respiratoires*, vol. 27, no. 7, pp. 693–702, 2010.

[105] C. Bogardus, S. Lillioja, D. Mott, C. Hollenbeck, and G. Reaven, "Relationship between degree of obesity and in vivo insulin action in man," *American Journal of Physiology-Endocrinology And Metabolism*, vol. 248, no. 3, pp. E286–E291, 1985.

[106] S. K. Gan, A. D. Kriketos, A. M. Poynten, S. M. Furler, C. H. Thompson, E. W. Kraegen, L. V. Campbell, and D. J. Chisholm, "Insulin action, regional fat, and myocyte lipid: altered relationships with increased adiposity," *Obesity Research*, vol. 11, no. 11, pp. 1295–1305, 2003.

[107] J. Reinus and D. Simon, *Gastrointestinal Anatomy and Physiology.* Wiley Online Library, 2014.

[108] A. D. Cherrington, "Banting lecture 1997. control of glucose uptake and release by the liver in vivo," *Diabetes*, vol. 48, no. 5, pp. 1198–1214, 1999.

[109] K. Foster-Powell, S. H. Holt, and J. C. Brand-Miller, "International table of glycemic index and glycemic load values: 2002," *The American Journal of Clinical Nutrition*, vol. 76, no. 1, pp. 5–56, 2002.

[110] R. Thibault, N. Cano, and C. Pichard, "Quantification of lean tissue losses during cancer and hiv infection/aids," *Current Opinion in Clinical Nutrition & Metabolic Care*, vol. 14, no. 3, pp. 261–267, 2011.

[111] W. D. Leslie, N. Miller, L. Rogala, and C. N. Bernstein, "Body mass and composition affect bone density in recently diagnosed inflammatory

bowel disease: the manitoba ibd cohort study," *Inflammatory Bowel Diseases*, vol. 15, no. 1, pp. 39–46, 2009.

[112] R. Thibault and C. Pichard, "Nutrition and clinical outcome in intensive care patients," *Current Opinion in Clinical Nutrition & Metabolic Care*, vol. 13, no. 2, pp. 177–183, 2010.

[113] C. Pichard, U. G. Kyle, P. Jolliet, D. O. Slosman, T. Rochat, L. Nicod, J. Romand, N. Mensi, and J.-C. Chevrolet, "Treatment of cachexia with recombinant growth hormone in a patient before lung transplantation: a case report," *Critical Care Medicine*, vol. 27, no. 8, pp. 1639–1642, 1999.

[114] S. Antoun, V. Baracos, L. Birdsell, B. Escudier, and M. Sawyer, "Low body mass index and sarcopenia associated with dose-limiting toxicity of sorafenib in patients with renal cell carcinoma," *Annals of Oncology*, vol. 21, no. 8, pp. 1594–1598, 2010.

[115] C. M. Prado, V. E. Baracos, L. J. McCargar, M. Mourtzakis, K. E. Mulder, T. Reiman, C. A. Butts, A. G. Scarfe, and M. B. Sawyer, "Body composition as an independent determinant of 5-fluorouracil–based chemotherapy toxicity," *Clinical Cancer Research*, vol. 13, no. 11, pp. 3264–3268, 2007.

[116] P. Arpaia, F. Clemente, and A. Zanesco, "Low-invasive diagnosis of metallic prosthesis osseointegration by electrical impedance spectroscopy," *IEEE Transactions on Instrumentation and Measurement*, vol. 56, no. 3, pp. 784–789, 2007.

[117] B. Tsai, H. Xue, E. Birgersson, S. Ollmar, and U. Birgersson, "Analysis of a mechanistic model for non-invasive bioimpedance of intact skin," *Journal of Electrical Bioimpedance*, vol. 8, no. 1, pp. 84–96, 2017.

[118] T. Yoshida, W.-C. Kim, K. Kawamoto, T. Hirashima, Y. Oka, and T. Kubo, "Measurement of bone electrical impedance in fracture healing," *Journal of Orthopaedic Science*, vol. 14, no. 3, pp. 320–329, 2009.

[119] M. C. Lin, *Impedance Spectroscopy for Surface and Fracture Wounds: Sensor Development and Clinical Application.* PhD thesis, UCSF, 2018.

[120] M. S. Roberts, S. Cross, and Y. Anissimov, "Factors affecting the formation of a skin reservoir for topically applied solutes," *Skin Pharmacology and Physiology*, vol. 17, no. 1, pp. 3–16, 2004.

[121] H. Lukaski, "Regional bioelectrical impedance analysis: applications in health and medicine," *Acta Diabetologica*, vol. 40, no. 1, pp. s196–s199, 2003.

[122] L. Maxey and J. Magnusson, *Rehabilitation for the postsurgical orthopedic patient.* Elsevier Health Sciences, 2013.

[123] J. Ekstrand, M. Hägglund, and M. Waldén, "Epidemiology of muscle injuries in professional football (soccer)," *The American Journal of Sports Medicine*, vol. 39, no. 6, pp. 1226–1232, 2011.

[124] V. Francavilla, T. Bongiovanni, F. Genovesi, P. Minafra, and G. Francavilla, "Localized bioelectrical impedance analysis: how useful is it in the follow-up of muscle injury," *Med Sport*, vol. 68, pp. 323–34, 2015.

[125] E. M. Bartels, E. R. Sørensen, and A. P. Harrison, "Multi-frequency bioimpedance in human muscle assessment," *Physiological Reports*, vol. 3, no. 4, p. e12354, 2015.

[126] A. Liao, M. C. Lin, L. C. Ritz, S. L. Swisher, D. Ni, K. Mann, Y. Khan, S. Roy, M. R. Harrison, A. C. Arias, *et al.*, "Impedance sensing device for monitoring ulcer healing in human patients," in *2015 37th Annual International Conference of the IEEE Engineering in Medicine and Biology Society (EMBC)*, pp. 5130–5133, IEEE, 2015.

[127] S. Hersek, H. Töreyin, C. N. Teague, M. L. Millard-Stafford, H.-K. Jeong, M. M. Bavare, P. Wolkoff, M. N. Sawka, and O. T. Inan, "Wearable vector electrical bioimpedance system to assess knee joint health," *IEEE Transactions on Biomedical Engineering*, vol. 64, no. 10, pp. 2353–2360, 2016.

[128] S. Hersek, H. Töreyin, and O. T. Inan, "A robust system for longitudinal knee joint edema and blood flow assessment based on vector bioimpedance measurements," *IEEE Transactions on Biomedical Circuits and Systems*, vol. 10, no. 3, pp. 545–555, 2015.

[129] C. Pichonnaz, J.-P. Bassin, D. Currat, E. Martin, and B. M. Jolles, "Bioimpedance for oedema evaluation after total knee arthroplasty," *Physiotherapy Research International*, vol. 18, no. 3, pp. 140–147, 2013.

[130] A. H. Dell'Osa, C. J. Felice, and F. Simini, "Bioimpedance and bone fracture detection: A state of the art," in *Journal of Physics: Conference Series*, vol. 1272, p. 012010, IOP Publishing, 2019.

[131] C. Gabriel, "Compilation of the dielectric properties of body tissues at rf and microwave frequencies.," tech. rep., KING'S COLL LONDON (UNITED KINGDOM) DEPT OF PHYSICS, 1996.

[132] J. Sierpowska, M. Hakulinen, J. Töyräs, J. Day, H. Weinans, I. Kiviranta, J. Jurvelin, and R. Lappalainen, "Interrelationships between electrical properties and microstructure of human trabecular bone," *Physics in Medicine & Biology*, vol. 51, no. 20, p. 5289, 2006.

[133] S. Saha and P. A. Williams, "Comparison of the electrical and dielectric behavior of wet human cortical and cancellous bone tissue from the distal tibia," *Journal of Orthopaedic Research*, vol. 13, no. 4, pp. 524–532, 1995.

[134] S. Kumaravel, "Monitoring of fracture healing by electrical conduction: A new diagnostic procedure," *Indian Journal of Orthopaedics*, vol. 46, pp. 384–390, 2012.

[135] O. M. Steihaug, B. Bogen, M. H. Kristoffersen, and A. H. Ranhoff, "Bones, blood and steel: How bioelectrical impedance analysis is affected by hip fracture and surgical implants," *Journal of Electrical Bioimpedance*, vol. 8, no. 1, pp. 54–59, 2017.

[136] P. Arpaia, V. Bruno, F. Clemente, and A. Zanesco, "Low-invasive diagnosis of prothesis osseointegration by electrical impedance spectroscopy," in *2005 IEEE Instrumentationand Measurement Technology Conference Proceedings*, vol. 2, pp. 929–933, IEEE, 2005.

[137] P. Arpaia, F. Clemente, and C. Romanucci, "Impedance spectroscopy-based measurement of cochlear prosthesis osseointegration: in-vivo test procedure and characterization," *Proc. of IMTC 2007*, pp. 1–3, 2007.

[138] E. B. Neves, A. V. Pino, R. M. V. R. De Almeida, and M. N. De Souza, "Knee bioelectric impedance assessment in healthy/with osteoarthritis subjects," *Physiological Measurement*, vol. 31, no. 2, p. 207, 2009.

[139] J. Hadgraft, "Passive enhancement strategies in topical and transdermal drug delivery," *International Journal of Pharmaceutics*, vol. 184, no. 1, pp. 1–6, 1999.

[140] H. Trommer and R. Neubert, "Overcoming the stratum corneum: the modulation of skin penetration," *Skin Pharmacology and Physiology*, vol. 19, no. 2, pp. 106–121, 2006.

[141] C. Herkenne, A. Naik, Y. N. Kalia, J. Hadgraft, and R. H. Guy, "Dermatopharmacokinetic prediction of topical drug bioavailability in vivo," *Journal of Investigative Dermatology*, vol. 127, no. 4, pp. 887–894, 2007.

[142] C. Herkenne, I. Alberti, A. Naik, Y. N. Kalia, F.-X. Mathy, V. Préat, and R. H. Guy, "In vivo methods for the assessment of topical drug bioavailability," *Pharmaceutical Research*, vol. 25, no. 1, p. 87, 2008.

[143] P. Arpaia, U. Cesaro, and N. Moccaldi, "Measuring the drug absorbed by biological tissues in laboratory emulation of dermatological topical treatments," in *2016 IEEE International Symposium on Medical Measurements and Applications (MeMeA)*, pp. 1–5, IEEE, 2016.

[144] E. N. Marieb and K. Hoehn, *Human anatomy & physiology.* Pearson education, 2007.

[145] B. Rigaud, J.-P. Morucci, and N. Chauveau, "Bioelectrical impedance techniques in medicine part i: bioimpedance measurement second section: impedance spectrometry," *Critical Reviews^{TM} in Biomedical Engineering*, vol. 24, no. 4-6, 1996.

[146] L. Wu, Y. Ogawa, and A. Tagawa, "Electrical impedance spectroscopy analysis of eggplant pulp and effects of drying and freezing–thawing treatments on its impedance characteristics," *Journal of Food Engineering*, vol. 87, no. 2, pp. 274–280, 2008.

[147] I. E. Commission, *IEC 60601-2-33 Medical Electrical Equipment-Part I*, vol. 2. 2001.

[148] "Solartron 1260a impedance analyzer https://www.ameteksi.com/products/frequency-response-analyzers/1260a-impedance-gain-phase-analyzer." Accessed: 2021-07-05.

[149] "Fiab pg500 disposable gelled electrodes." Accessed: 2021-06-28.

[150] U. Birgersson, E. Birgersson, and S. Ollmar, "Estimating electrical properties and the thickness of skin with electrical impedance spectroscopy: Mathematical analysis and measurements," *Journal of Electrical Bioimpedance*, vol. 3, no. 1, pp. 51–60, 2019.

[151] "Agilent 4263b lcr meter. https://www.keysight.com/it/en/product/4263b/lcr-meter-100-hz-to-100-khz.html." Accessed: 2020-02-28.

[152] P. De Bièvre, "The 2012 international vocabulary of metrology: "vim"," *Accreditation and Quality Assurance*, vol. 17, no. 2, pp. 231–232, 2012.

[153] U. Birgersson, E. Birgersson, P. Åberg, I. Nicander, and S. Ollmar, "Non-invasive bioimpedance of intact skin: mathematical modeling and experiments," *Physiological Measurement*, vol. 32, no. 1, p. 1, 2010.

[154] M. E. Valentinuzzi, "Bioelectrical impedance techniques in medicine part i: Bioimpedance measurement first section: General concepts," *Critical Reviews^{TM} in Biomedical Engineering*, vol. 24, no. 4-6, 1996.

[155] D. C. Montgomery and G. C. Runger, *Applied statistics and probability for engineers.* John Wiley & Sons, 2010.

[156] M. S. Phadke, *Quality engineering using robust design.* Prentice Hall, NJ, 1989.

[157] P. Ross, *Taguchi techniques for quality engineering.* Mc Graw-Hill, 1996.

[158] F. P. Schmook, J. G. Meingassner, and A. Billich, "Comparison of human skin or epidermis models with human and animal skin in in-vitro percutaneous absorption," *International Journal of Pharmaceutics*, vol. 215, no. 1, pp. 51–56, 2001.

[159] J. E. Seto, B. E. Polat, R. F. Lopez, D. Blankschtein, and R. Langer, "Effects of ultrasound and sodium lauryl sulfate on the transdermal delivery of hydrophilic permeants: Comparative in vitro studies with full-thickness and split-thickness pig and human skin," *Journal of Controlled Release*, vol. 145, no. 1, pp. 26–32, 2010.

[160] N. Sekkat, Y. N. Kalia, and R. H. Guy, "Biophysical study of porcine ear skin in vitro and its comparison to human skin in vivo," *Journal of Pharmaceutical Sciences*, vol. 91, no. 11, pp. 2376–2381, 2002.

[161] D. Carney and F. Leng, "What do you mean by cots? finally, a useful answer," *IEEE software*, vol. 17, no. 2, pp. 83–86, 2000.

[162] A. D. Inch., "Eval-aducm350 evaluation board; http://www.analog.com/en/design-center/evaluation-hardware-and-software/evaluation-boards-kits/eval-aducm350.html."

[163] "Arm cortex-m3." Accessed: 2021-04-16.

[164] A. Basu, S. Dube, M. Slama, I. Errazuriz, J. C. Amezcua, Y. C. Kudva, T. Peyser, R. E. Carter, C. Cobelli, and R. Basu, "Time lag of glucose from intravascular to interstitial compartment in humans," *Diabetes*, vol. 62, no. 12, pp. 4083–4087, 2013.

[165] B. Shashaj, E. Busetto, and N. Sulli, "Benefits of a bolus calculator in pre-and postprandial glycaemic control and meal flexibility of paediatric patients using continuous subcutaneous insulin infusion (csii)," *Diabetic Medicine*, vol. 25, no. 9, pp. 1036–1042, 2008.

[166] R. J. Young, W. J. Hannan, B. M. Frier, J. M. Steel, and L. J. Duncan, "Diabetic lipohypertrophy delays insulin absorption," *Diabetes Care*, vol. 7, no. 5, pp. 479–480, 1984.

[167] T. S. Morley, J. Y. Xia, and P. E. Scherer, "Selective enhancement of insulin sensitivity in the mature adipocyte is sufficient for systemic metabolic improvements," *Nature Communications*, vol. 6, no. 1, pp. 1–11, 2015.

[168] S.-C. Chow, "Bioavailability and bioequivalence in drug development," *Wiley Interdisciplinary Reviews: Computational Statistics*, vol. 6, no. 4, pp. 304–312, 2014.

[169] C. Cobelli, E. Renard, and B. Kovatchev, "Artificial pancreas: past, present, future," *Diabetes*, vol. 60, no. 11, pp. 2672–2682, 2011.

[170] C. Tan, S. Liu, J. Jia, and F. Dong, "A wideband electrical impedance tomography system based on sensitive bioimpedance spectrum bandwidth," *IEEE Transactions on Instrumentation and Measurement*, vol. 69, no. 1, pp. 144–154, 2019.

[171] J.-J. Cabrera-López and J. Velasco-Medina, "Structured approach and impedance spectroscopy microsystem for fractional-order electrical characterization of vegetable tissues," *IEEE Transactions on Instrumentation and Measurement*, vol. 69, no. 2, pp. 469–478, 2019.

[172] G. Annuzzi, P. Arpaia, U. Cesaro, O. Cuomo, M. Frosolone, S. Grassini, N. Moccaldi, and I. Sannino, "A customized bioimpedance meter for monitoring insulin bioavailability," in *2020 IEEE International Instrumentation and Measurement Technology Conference (I2MTC)*, pp. 1–5, IEEE, 2020.

[173] A. Devices, "Aducm350 datasheet and product info; https://www.analog.com/media/en/technical-documentation/data-sheets/aducm350.pdf,"

[174] D. S. Jevsevar, P. B. Shores, K. Mullen, D. M. Schulte, G. A. Brown, and D. S. Cummins, "Mixed treatment comparisons for nonsurgical treatment of knee osteoarthritis: a network meta-analysis," *JAAOS-Journal of the American Academy of Orthopaedic Surgeons*, vol. 26, no. 9, pp. 325–336, 2018.

[175] S. Derry, P. Conaghan, J. A. P. Da Silva, P. J. Wiffen, and R. A. Moore, "Topical nsaids for chronic musculoskeletal pain in adults," *Cochrane Database of Systematic Reviews*, no. 4, 2016.

[176] F. Rannou, J.-P. Pelletier, and J. Martel-Pelletier, "Efficacy and safety of topical nsaids in the management of osteoarthritis: evidence from real-life setting trials and surveys," in *Seminars in Arthritis and Rheumatism*, vol. 45, pp. S18–S21, Elsevier, 2016.

[177] P. Clarys, K. Alewaeters, R. Lambrecht, and A. Barel, "Skin color measurements: comparison between three instruments: the chromameter®, the dermaspectrometer® and the mexameter®," *Skin Research and Technology*, vol. 6, no. 4, pp. 230–238, 2000.

[178] K. M. Deligiannidis, N. Byatt, and M. P. Freeman, "Pharmacotherapy for mood disorders in pregnancy: a review of pharmacokinetic changes and clinical recommendations for therapeutic drug monitoring," *Journal of Clinical Psychopharmacology*, vol. 34, no. 2, p. 244, 2014.

[179] V. P. Shah, G. L. Flynn, A. Yacobi, H. I. Maibach, C. Bon, N. M. Fleischer, T. J. Franz, S. A. Kaplan, J. Kawamoto, L. J. Lesko, *et al.*, "Bioequivalence of topical dermatological dosage forms–methods of evaluation of bioequivalence," *Skin Pharmacology and Physiology*, vol. 11, no. 2, pp. 117–124, 1998.

[180] R. Sanz, A. C. Calpena, M. Mallandrich, and B. Clares, "Enhancing topical analgesic administration: review and prospect for transdermal and transbuccal drug delivery systems.," *Current Pharmaceutical Design*, vol. 21, no. 20, pp. 2867–2882, 2015.

[181] S. Grassini, S. Corbellini, E. Angelini, F. Ferraris, and M. Parvis, "Low-cost impedance spectroscopy system based on a logarithmic amplifier,"

IEEE Transactions on Instrumentation and Measurement, vol. 64, no. 5, pp. 1110–1117, 2014.

[182] J. Zuo, L. Du, M. Li, B. Liu, W. Zhu, and Y. Jin, "Transdermal enhancement effect and mechanism of iontophoresis for non-steroidal anti-inflammatory drugs," *International Journal of Pharmaceutics*, vol. 466, no. 1-2, pp. 76–82, 2014.

[183] E. Yelin, S. Weinstein, and T. King, "The burden of musculoskeletal diseases in the united states," in *Seminars in arthritis and rheumatism*, vol. 46, pp. 259–260, 2016.

[184] J. F. Abulhasan and M. J. Grey, "Anatomy and physiology of knee stability," *Journal of Functional Morphology and Kinesiology*, vol. 2, no. 4, p. 34, 2017.

[185] A. Dodds, C. Halewood, C. Gupte, A. Williams, and A. Amis, "The anterolateral ligament: anatomy, length changes and association with the segond fracture," *The Bone & Joint Journal*, vol. 96, no. 3, pp. 325–331, 2014.

[186] R. F. LaPrade, A. H. Engebretsen, T. V. Ly, S. Johansen, F. A. Wentorf, and L. Engebretsen, "The anatomy of the medial part of the knee," *JBJS*, vol. 89, no. 9, pp. 2000–2010, 2007.

[187] B. Medical, "Medical gallery of blausen medical 2014," *Wiki Journal of Medicine*, vol. 1, no. 2, pp. 1–79, 2014.

[188] K. S. Cole and R. H. Cole, "Dispersion and absorption in dielectrics i. alternating current characteristics," *The Journal of Chemical Physics*, vol. 9, no. 4, pp. 341–351, 1941.

[189] A. Kraszewski, M. A. Stuchly, and S. S. Stuchly, "Ana calibration method for measurements of dielectric properties," *IEEE Transactions on Instrumentation and Measurement*, vol. 32, no. 2, pp. 385–387, 1983.

[190] M.-R. Tofighi and A. S. Daryoush, "Biological tissue complex permittivity measured from $s\_\{21\}$—error analysis and error reduction by reference measurements," *IEEE Transactions on Instrumentation and Measurement*, vol. 58, no. 7, pp. 2316–2327, 2009.

[191] D. Miklavčič, N. Pavšelj, and F. X. Hart, "Electric properties of tissues," *Wiley encyclopedia of Biomedical Engineering*, 2006.

[192] A. R. Dabrowska, S. Derler, F. Spano, M. Camenzind, and Annaheim, "Materials used to simulate physical properties of human skin," *Skin Research and Technology*, vol. 22, no. 1, pp. 3–14, 2016.

[193] U. Birgersson, E. Birgersson, I. Nicander, and S. Ollmar, "A methodology for extracting the electrical properties of human skin," *Physiological Measurement*, vol. 34, no. 6, p. 723, 2013.

[194] F. A. Duck, *Physical properties of tissues: a comprehensive reference book*. Academic press, 2013.

[195] P. Oltulu, B. Ince, N. Kökbudak, F. Kılıç, *et al.*, "Measurement of epidermis, dermis, and total skin thicknesses from six different body regions with a new ethical histometric technique," *Türk Plastik, Rekonstrüktif ve Estetik Cerrahi Dergisi (Turk J Plast Surg)*, vol. 26, no. 2, pp. 56–61, 2018.

[196] J. Sandby-Moller, T. Poulsen, and H. C. Wulf, "Epidermal thickness at different body sites: relationship to age, gender, pigmentation, blood content, skin type and smoking habits," *Acta Dermato Venereologica*, vol. 83, no. 6, pp. 410–413, 2003.

[197] R. R. Warner, M. C. Myers, and D. A. Taylor, "Electron probe analysis of human skin: determination of the water concentration profile.," *Journal of Investigative Dermatology*, vol. 90, no. 2, pp. 218–224, 1988.

[198] N. Nakagawa, M. Matsumoto, and S. Sakai, "In vivo measurement of the water content in the dermis by confocal raman spectroscopy," *Skin Research and Technology*, vol. 16, no. 2, pp. 137–141, 2010.

[199] B. Nadeem, R. Bacha, and S. A. Gilani, "Correlation of subcutaneous fat measured on ultrasound with body mass index," *Journal of Medical ultrasound*, vol. 26, no. 4, p. 205, 2018.

[200] G. Anastasi, *Trattato di anatomia umana*. Edi. Ermes, 2007.

[201] M. Douglas, A. Anderson, and E. Michelle, "Mosby's medical, nursing, & allied health dictionary," *Padova: Piccin*, 2004.

[202] W. J. Hamilton, *Textbook of human anatomy*. Springer, 1982.

[203] B. Epstein and K. Foster, "Anisotropy in the dielectric properties of skeletal muscle," *Medical and Biological Engineering and Computing*, vol. 21, no. 1, p. 51, 1983.

[204] R. Aaron, M. Huang, and C. Shiffman, "Anisotropy of human muscle via non-invasive impedance measurements," *Physics in Medicine & Biology*, vol. 42, no. 7, p. 1245, 1997.

[205] S. Čorović, A. Županič, S. Kranjc, B. Al Sakere, A. Leroy-Willig, L. M. Mir, and D. Miklavčič, "The influence of skeletal muscle anisotropy on electroporation: in vivo study and numerical modeling," *Medical & biological Engineering & Computing*, vol. 48, no. 7, pp. 637–648, 2010.

[206] C. Lefrou, P. Fabry, and J.-C. Poignet, *Electrochemistry: the basics, with examples.* Springer Science & Business Media, 2012.

[207] J. D. Barrett, "Taguchi's quality engineering handbook," *Technometrics*, 2012.

[208] M. Silvestre, A. Saeed, R. Cervera, and Escriba, "Rabbit and pig ear skin sample cryobanking: effects of storage time and temperature of the whole ear extirpated immediately after death," *Theriogenology*, vol. 59, no. 5, pp. 1469–1477, 2003.

[209] S. G. Danby, "Biological variation in skin barrier function: from a (atopic dermatitis) to x (xerosis)," *Skin Barrier Function*, vol. 49, pp. 47–60, 2016.

[210] D. M. Olsson and L. S. Nelson, "The nelder-mead simplex procedure for function minimization," *Technometrics*, vol. 17, no. 1, pp. 45–51, 1975.

Index

Milton Keynes UK
Ingram Content Group UK Ltd.
UKHW021843301123
433521UK00003B/10

9 780367 765989